Looking on the Bright Side
A Vet's Tale

—

Sue Devereux

To the staff of Salisbury District Hospital past and present, without whom I would not be here.

All profits from the sale of this book will be donated to the Stars Appeal, the NHS charity for Salisbury District Hospital—a small thank you for saving my life at least twice.

CONTENTS

PROLOGUE

The surgeon walked back into the room and looked me straight in the eye. 'The results will be back in a week but expect bad news.' For once I was speechless but in my mind there was just one question: 'How bad?'

I'd seen the speckled deposits of calcium on the scan and the X-ray so I knew I had cancer and was about to embark on a path along which I had no desire to travel. That was five weeks ago. Today I have just woken up from the anaesthetic and in another two weeks when the results come through, I will have the answer...

For now I can only wonder about the future and hope I have one. As I lie here, still sleepy and entrusting my care to the capable hands of the brilliant hospital team, I look back at my career as a veterinary surgeon and know that whatever happens, I have no regrets.

PART ONE

LOOKING ON THE BRIGHT SIDE

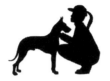

I have always been an optimist. When I qualified as a vet in 1983, there were very few job vacancies. I dreamt of being a country vet in the South of England but the sceptics told me that there was no chance of that. Female? Large animal work? Southern location? 'Get real; take a small animal job and treat dogs and cats,' I was repeatedly advised.

One year on I was living my dream. I remember driving past Badbury Rings on a late September afternoon and being spellbound by the enchanting beauty created by the still-warm sun on the landscape. The trees formed an archway over the road through which the dazzling light cascaded in rivulets and pools. The green leaves shimmered in the breeze and beyond the old and twisted trunks I could see the fallow and fertile fields stretched out on the horizon.

I pulled off the road and climbed to the top of Badbury Rings with the cool breeze ruffling my hair. I huddled into my Barbour coat and surveyed the tranquil scene around me. Seagulls gathered on the rich, bare earth and in the distance, I could make out the point-to-point course where I had picnicked with my farming friends earlier in the year, full of cheer despite the relentless rain.

As I sat on the hilltop, absorbing the solitude and peacefulness, I remembered vividly coming to Wimborne for an interview, full of hope and the promise of an exciting and rewarding future as a vet. I was greeted with the smiling, friendly face of Tim, one of the two partners in the practice. He was not completely unknown to me. Many years before, I had attended his wedding when he married the elder sister of my best friend at school. Little did we know then how our futures would be entwined.

Tim showed me around the premises and I was at once impressed by the facilities. The advertisement in the *Veterinary Record* made it subtly clear that they were hoping to find an experienced male vet, preferably married and with a wife to answer the telephone. And here I was, still doing my final exams, full of enthusiasm but no experience, single and female.

We sat in the waiting room and chatted for a while. All the time I felt there was at least a little hope of success as Tim kept saying, 'Your duties will be…,' and each time my heart took a great lurch. I was desperate to be given a chance and yet terrified of how I would cope if I were. Chris, the young assistant who had been with the practice for three years, then joined us. I realised I had met him before and at that moment he felt like a long-lost friend. Perhaps he would be on my side.

It was a hot, sticky summer afternoon and a short, rather stocky man came into the waiting room. Wearing shorts and a torn shirt, and looking rather warm but jolly, he left a trail of hay and straw on the floor behind him. I wondered who this was and was mildly surprised when he was introduced as Richard, the other partner. Unbeknown to me I had just met the man who would be my guide and mentor through my first years in veterinary practice and who remains my friend today.

As the sun dipped behind the horizon, I wondered what the future would hold. So many crossroads and pathways were to open up before me.

2

THE ADVENTURE BEGINS

To my absolute delight and joy, I got the job. I later learnt that I was their second choice but the other candidate turned it down as the salary was too low. If they only knew, I would have done it for nothing!

The early days in practice can have a big influence on your career. It is so important to be able to ask for advice and discuss any difficult cases without being made to feel incompetent. To help me settle in, Mr Birrell, the retired senior partner, came back to work for a few weeks. I remember with great affection him beckoning me over to the day book where the nurses wrote down all the visits, and going through the list. 'Now which of these do you feel you could tackle?' he would ask kindly and then send me off with a few words of advice.

What an adventurous journey I was beginning. I had wanted to work in a mixed practice to become competent at treating a wide range of animals, and indeed the variety was just amazing. When the phone rang at night, I never knew whether it would be for a cow, horse, sheep, goat, pig, dog, cat, budgie, rabbit or mouse, to name but a few.

And night duty seemed to happen very often. With Chris

now invited to be a partner, that was one night each for the men and four for me. The upside was that I very quickly tackled all the scary emergencies that new graduates face and got them safely behind me. In any case, I never felt completely alone because as we left the practice after evening surgery each night, Richard would always mention in conversation his evening plans. It was his way of letting me know where he was if I needed any help, which was wonderfully reassuring.

There were times when I went to emergencies and realised that no one had ever taught me how to deal with that particular situation. I remember worrying about a cow that had torn her tongue on a barbed-wire fence. It was partially severed and too dirty to suture. What should I do? I trimmed off the damaged tissue, cleaned it up and gave her antibiotics and painkillers. Looking back, that was the right thing to do. The truth is that the tongue would heal and she would manage to eat perfectly well, or it would not and she would have to be slaughtered. At the time though I felt I had not done enough but thankfully she made a good recovery.

The two nurses, Christine and Tanya also supported me in those early days with patience and wisdom, especially in the operating theatre. When the uterus of the cat I was trying to spay was mysteriously elusive, I remember Christine advising me that in this situation, the other vets might enlarge the incision. Of course!

In such a busy practice, there was little time for much else apart from work. But in the summer evenings when I was free, I would drive to Sunnylands Farm and take my horse Lucy out for a ride. Hacking through the beautiful Dorset countryside was a delightful way to relax at the end of the day. I had persuaded my father to lend me the money to buy a horse whilst I was a student and it was a joke between us that I paid him back just 50 pence each month. In order to earn the money for Lucy's keep, I'd had various jobs when I went home for the holidays. In the mornings and evenings, I milked a small herd of Jersey cows and in the afternoon, I groomed for a family with show ponies. It gave me huge pleasure when I qualified as a vet to be able to keep Lucy in a lovely setting with everything she needed, rather than living out all year in a field surrounded by busy Bristol traffic.

Then I would stop at the fish and chip shop in Corfe Mullen on the way home and buy whatever they had left. Sometimes when I was very late, they would slip something extra into the bag so it was not wasted. I fondly remember all those little acts of kindness.

Back then I had very few possessions and lived in a rented house. I came home one evening to find a young man from the Veterinary Insurance Agency waiting patiently on my doorstep. I was obviously on his list of new graduates and therefore a potential customer. I think even he was surprised when after I'd given him a cup of tea, we made a list of my belongings: one sleeping bag, one old cushion (my pillow), a second-hand record player and a few clothes. To his credit he kept a completely straight face and quoted me a premium of just a couple of pounds, which I accepted.

It was in those early days that I decided to buy a puppy for company. The owner of the house agreed that I could have a small dog, but not the golden retriever that I really wanted. So one evening I set off with one of the nurses to select a Cavalier King Charles Spaniel puppy and came back with two. Twiggy was a blenheim bitch and Poppy was tricolour. They were from different litters but bonded immediately and from day one came to work with me in a big cardboard box on the back seat of my car. I remember at the end of that evening having just £25 left in my bank account, but it was money well spent as the dogs gave me eleven and sixteen years respectively of love and friendship.

3

NEW FRIENDS

Talking of friends, I didn't have any to start with. I was simply too busy enjoying my work and loving it. Until I met Jayne, that is, when life became even more fun.

Jayne first called me out to do a pre-purchase examination of a horse she was hoping to buy. This is a very thorough examination taking about an hour and a half to ensure as far as possible that the horse is in good health and suitable for its intended purpose.

Unfortunately for Jayne, the first horse was lame; the second had a respiratory complaint and the third, although only four years old, was already showing signs of wear and tear on his limbs, indicating that he would probably not stand up to the rigours of one-day eventing.

As part of the examination, the vet performs flexion tests which involve holding up each limb in turn in a flexed position for about a minute then asking the horse to trot off, thus testing for any stiffness or lameness. On this very hot day, I had struggled with the excited and uncooperative colt and was hot and exhausted by the end of yet another examination with a disappointing outcome. It was now lunchtime and Jayne took one look at me and suggested we went to the pub for a cool drink. I declined at once as I had other visits to do but she pointed out that I had only taken half of the time allotted for the vetting and in any case we were 40 miles from the practice and no one was ever going to know (till now, that is).

As we chatted over a welcome ice-cold coke, Jayne enquired how I was settling in and what I did in my spare time. Work, ride, eat and sleep was too solitary, she decided, and from that moment she took me under her wing and set about introducing me to a lovely group of friends. That was the beginning of a summer of barbecues, supper parties and picnics. I made some lifelong friends and began to feel really at home in every way.

Other people who made a difference were Joan and Arthur, my school friend Sue's parents who now lived in an annexe attached to Tim's house. They had been very good friends with my parents when we lived just a few houses apart in Surrey. I had grown up knowing them and even lived with them whilst in the sixth form at school when my parents moved to Jersey. It was lovely to be able to drop in unannounced and be welcomed with a cup of tea and piece of cake, then to sit and either reminisce, excitedly share a story about my day or even to have a moan about Tim being too bossy.

I also made many friends amongst the farmers and their dairymen. It tickled me pink that more often than not they did not recognise their vet at parties in a sparkly dress and pretty shoes. Wellies, waterproof trousers and a calving gown with an aroma of cow muck were my more familiar attire. Which reminds me of my sister Jane's wedding. I was still a student, lambing ewes in the Dorset hills with my friend Claire from vet school. We worked all hours in all weathers, loving the thrill of welcoming new life and caring for the lambs in their early days. My mother was taking no chances and insisted I arrive in

Cambridge a day early so she could supervise my haircut and the purchase of a suitable outfit. She honestly thought I would turn up in green waterproofs and wellies.

4

SCARY EMERGENCIES

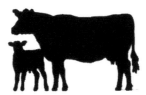

There are two 'first times' that really stand out in my memory and both were caesareans. Every time I was called back to the surgery to attend a whelping bitch, I would dash into the operating theatre and quickly read through my university surgery notes. These events always seemed to occur in the evenings when I was on my own, apart from the wonderful nurses, that is.

By now I had spayed quite a number of bitches and in theory a caesarean was no more difficult, but it would be a relief to tackle my first. There were three false alarms when I was able to deliver the puppies without surgery, but then came the call I will never forget.

A gentleman rang in great distress to say that his Jack Russell was in difficulty but another practice had refused to operate as he could not pay for the treatment. Well there was no doubt that this was meant to come to me. As he walked through the door with the beautiful little dog in his arms, she looked at me with her big brown eyes and a tiny wag of her tail. He put her onto the table and she was perfectly mannered whilst I gently examined her. After establishing that she could not give birth naturally, I asked him if there was any chance he would be able to pay off the bill at £10 a month and he smiled in relief and said that would not be a problem. Of course, I would have gone ahead anyway (even if the cost was deducted from my wages!)

It was probably one of the easiest and most satisfying operations I have ever performed. The Jack Russell was co-operative to anaesthetise and everything went according to plan. Just an hour later, I rang the gentleman and asked him to come and collect her and the five healthy, strong pups.

As I handed him the cardboard box with the little dog and the puppies on a warm pad, he burst into tears and told me that earlier that night his eight-year-old son had gone to bed distraught, believing his dog would have to be put to sleep. Now he was going to have a lovely surprise and he could not thank me enough. Even the memory brings goosebumps to my arms. I felt so happy that I was able to help and the circumstances made the experience extra special.

My second caesarean was completely different. Every now and again at the practice there would be an urgent shout for Richard to come to the phone to speak to a particular farmer. Not understanding the air of urgency these calls always evoked, I asked the nurses if there was a problem. 'Oh yes,' they said. 'This man is always difficult and will only speak to Richard. He won't let any of the other vets visit his farm.'

Imagine then my thoughts when on a Saturday afternoon three weeks later, a call came through for a calving on this very farm with the message that it was likely to be a caesarean. The farm was on the outskirts of our practice area, miles away, and of course I had not been there before so would have to find it first. The nurses who answered the phone didn't tell me what the response was when the farmer learnt that I was on my way, probably just as well. I loaded the kit into the car and everything else that I could possibly need and set off. These days caesareans are often performed with two vets in attendance but in 1983 you just got on and did the job alone.

The butterflies in my tummy were intense as I set out, but in a way it wasn't so bad because the man was going to be unhappy with the new 'girl vet' coming anyway, so if I ran into problems and had to call for assistance it was probably better to happen there than anywhere else as I was unlikely to do any further work for him.

Three stern-faced, silent men greeted me. In a way that was good news—plenty of help. Furthermore, the heifer was tied up ready in a well-lit barn with a clean, deep straw bed. Better still she was a tiny little thing that had accidentally been served by a large Belgian Blue bull, so it was recognised from the outset that there was no way she could deliver the huge calf naturally. These operations have a much greater chance of success if surgery is performed without the animal being subjected to uncomfortable and unsuccessful attempts to deliver the calf first. The final stroke of good luck was that as she had put all her energy into producing the calf, she was on the thin side, making all the bony landmarks for giving the local anaesthetic easy to find.

Whilst the anaesthetic was taking effect, she stood quietly as we clipped the hair from her flank and cleaned the skin ready for the operation. Suddenly all my nerves were gone as I focused on the task of delivering a live calf from this quiet and patient heifer. I was satisfied that her side was completely numb as I made my incisions through the skin, then the muscles and finally the womb wall. I positioned the calf so the men could grasp her legs and pull her gently out and onto the straw. She was so heavy that it took two of them to lift her and to our combined joy and relief, she shook her head and began to breathe.

Thirty minutes later the heifer was all stitched up and happily licking and bonding with her calf. With the ice broken, I was offered a cup of tea and we sat and watched them for a while. Then I packed up all the kit and made my way back to Wimborne with a real sense of accomplishment and relief. Another 'first' was safely behind me.

5

A HELPING HAND

I t isn't every day that you meet a knight in shining armour. I did one morning just three months after joining the practice. Quite a few young vets have minor car accidents, no doubt something to do with struggling to read the map (no satnav then) whilst looking at signposts and thinking about the imminent case.

I was on my way to visit a coughing pony. I quickly learnt that when people give directions over the phone, they tend to forget about all the gravel tracks leading nowhere when they tell you to take the third turning on the right.

It was not long before I realised that I had taken the wrong road as the trees became denser and the track was increasingly overgrown and then disappeared altogether. At least there was a convenient gateway to reverse into. Looking over my left shoulder, I swung slowly round and then to my amazement there was a most peculiar sensation as the back of the car dropped down and the front end seemed to rise in slow motion. As I opened the door, I was shocked to find just space beneath my feet. A six-foot-deep, concrete-lined drainage channel had become hidden under the vegetation and all that was stopping my car from dropping right into it was the exhaust pipe at the rear of the car. With a sense of horror as the vehicle rocked from side to side, I jumped to safety and wondered what the partners would say if they could see me and their car now.

It had just started to rain and I remembered with relief that there was a garage close by on the main road. Surely they would be able to help? Well apparently not. Two very unhelpful mechanics said there was nothing they could do and I should phone for a breakdown truck that would cost £100 and take quite a while to get there.

By now I was soaking wet and in rather a panic. I ran along the road, thinking I would have to get to a phone box, ring the practice and confess. Just then a white Range Rover coming towards me slowed down. As it pulled over, the electric window opened and a friendly voice asked, 'Is that your car back there in the ditch? Do you need any help?' The voice belonged to a blond man wearing a white shirt who looked kind. Breaking all the rules about never getting into a car with strangers, I gratefully jumped in.

After a good look at the car, my rescuer reckoned all we needed was a strong rope and he would be able to pull it out. I knew a large farm with two dairies that the practice looked after was just down the road. Now seemed like a good time to pay a visit and introduce myself. Oh well, I couldn't hope to get away with it altogether.

As we pulled up outside a large machinery shed, I found a tractor driver and explained my predicament. With no attempt to hide his amusement, he good-naturedly produced just what I needed. Ten minutes later my car was gently pulled back onto the track without even a scratch. I learnt my knight in shining armour was called Barry. He would not accept anything for his trouble and before driving away, he checked the car over for me and said not to worry about anything; he was just pleased to help.

I got to my next visit on time; no one had even missed me. Later in the day, I confessed to Chris who laughed and also decided that no harm had been done. But to this day, I remember with gratitude the kind man in the white Range Rover who appeared at a moment when I needed a helping hand.

6

THE OLD MAN

It was teatime on a summer afternoon when I was contacted on my car radio and asked to visit a retired farm worker on a large estate. From the directions that I received, I was rather uncertain of where to go but headed up the Cranborne road in the right general direction. Parts of the estate I knew well as the practice was very involved in the management of their two large dairies, but when I slowed my car and pulled off the main road under some trees and drove into a huge yard, I was venturing into new territory.

As I looked around, the place seemed to be deserted. I had parked on a huge expanse of concrete with smart large barns housing farm machinery and combine harvesters on one side and a tall brick and timber building to my left. The sun was very bright, making me squint. There was a concrete road leading off towards the pastures but otherwise the complex was shielded from the road and any other buildings by mature oak and beech trees.

I peered in through the closed windows to see storerooms and what looked as though it may be an office. No sign of the old gentleman. I wandered further along and found a door ajar that opened directly onto a steep flight of timber stairs. No one answered my shouts and I was about to give up when I caught sight of a thick piece of string dangling down from the left side of the wall at the foot of the stairs. Scrawled in pencil with an arrow pointing to the end of the string was the single word 'pull'. This I did and nothing happened. Where, I wondered, did the piece of string lead to? My eyes followed its course up the stairs, looped through a few hooks on the wall, disappearing around the corner at the top. Still not entirely sure that I had come to the right place and beginning to feel rather like an intruder, I gave the string a hard tug. After a pause of a couple of seconds, there was a faint tinkling sound. Then nothing.

At the point of giving up, I began to turn away but heard a door creak followed by the shuffling of footsteps. Not long afterwards an old man appeared at the top of the stairs wearing carpet slippers, baggy trousers and an old brown cardigan. 'You the vet?' he asked.

'Yes, I've come to see your dog.'

'Come on up then,' he said, turning away.

I hurried up the stairs and turned right onto what I presumed was a landing. It had no windows and was very dark. As I made my way towards the doorway at the far end, I had to squeeze between old iron beds and other furniture propped against the wall. The large room into which I followed the old gentleman made me feel as though I was entering another world and going back through time to the previous century.

Essentially the room was a huge attic. The walls were about five feet high with windows on two sides. The steeply pitched roof was supported by rafters and had a liberal coating of spiders' webs stretching between the beams. A giant wooden table completely covered by stacks of yellowing newspapers dating as far back as the 1930s took up the centre of the room. The back of the attic was in dark shadow but in the corner opposite the door was an old enamel sink. This room had no mains water or electricity but through a dusty, cracked window pane came a piece of pipe and several tendrils of ivy. The sunlight filtered into this corner of the room and reflected off a chipped white jug that collected run-off rainwater from the guttering outside. Laid out by the sink was a tea towel that had seen better days and a bar of soap in a blue and white china bowl.

As I glanced around, I realised that this home was a treasure trove of possessions and memories for my client. Old, curling photos and story books cluttered every available space amongst pieces of antique machinery and furniture. Some of the machinery was in pieces on the floor next to oily rags, obviously in the process of being repaired.

My eyes then rested on an ancient paraffin stove emitting a gentle, warm glow. Lying very close on a piece of carpet was a brown mongrel. This had to be my patient. He was seventeen years old and his eyes had a glazed, faraway look. Earlier in the day, he had experienced what sounded very much like a fit. But he was settled now, resting peacefully with his nose on his front paws. As I spoke quietly to him and gently began my examination, he opened both eyes without moving anything but his tail, which wagged three or four times as I stroked his head.

The little old dog had wasted away to a shadow of his former self and from the smell of his breath he was now in kidney failure. With glistening eyes the old man pulled over a wooden chair and sat down beside us. Since his wife died fifteen years ago, Gyp had been his best friend and whilst the man knew there was very little hope, he would like to keep the dog for one more day before having him put to sleep if there was nothing I could do. Knowing that he had to come to terms with the loss in his own way, I took a blood sample from the dog's forearm and injected him with some vitamins and anabolic steroids, promising to return the next day with the results.

I never did go back. The next morning my colleague Richard

told me that Gyp had experienced another fit during the evening whilst strolling around the yard and had been unable to climb back up the stairs. Richard had put him to sleep and helped the old man to bury him. He also told me that the gentleman was 88 years old and had worked on the farm since being a boy. No one had the heart to evict him when he retired; indeed, he had been offered a farm cottage but had turned it down in favour of the attic that had been his home for so many years.

Less than a month later, the old man passed away too.

7

TILLY

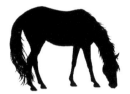

No one knew where Tilly came from. One day she just appeared, walking off a busy road into a smallholding that was home to three ponies, a few chickens and a goat. She seemed to know where she was going and walked straight into a stable that was all ready for the coming night. She took a deep drink of clean water from the filled bucket with great satisfaction and started to enjoy the sweet hay that was bursting out of the net in the corner.

When Lynne, the stable owner, came to bring her ponies in, she stared in disbelief at the thin, pot-bellied little mare that was now comfortably settled down for the night in the deep straw bed. Despite her obvious state of neglect, Tilly did not even get up during the commotion that her unexpected presence caused. Her soft brown eyes seemed to say, 'let me stay'.

A phone call to the police and neighbouring stables threw no light on Tilly's origins; no one had reported a missing pony.

The next morning everyone went off to a horse show and left a very happy Tilly wandering around the yard with access to her selected stable and a liberal supply of hay. She seemed to be enjoying the spring sunshine and showed no inclination to continue her travels.

It was just after lunch when Lynne's grandmother looked out of the kitchen window and saw the pony rolling on the muck heap. As she didn't have very much to do with the ponies, she thought very little of it until she noticed the pony was still there a couple of hours later. She put on her coat and cautiously moved closer until it became apparent that the little creature was in some kind of trouble. She walked quickly to the house and summoned some veterinary help.

When I arrived 25 minutes later, Tilly had gone back to 'her' stable and was lying down in the straw, sweating profusely. She stood up as I began my routine examination and my heart sank as I saw a second small black tail protruding from under her own. Not only was this mare foaling but she had one of the most difficult malpresentations to correct. In such a case, the aim is to push the foal back into the uterus and flex the hocks fully, allowing you to grasp the two hind feet one at a time and draw them outwards, whilst all the time protecting the womb with a cupped hand from being torn by the sharp little hooves.

By this stage the pony was already exhausted and had virtually given up. The foal was small and had obviously died so the task was to deliver it in a way to minimise the trauma and discomfort to the mare, who by now was not looking very good. Her dun coat was dark with sweat and her breathing fast and shallow. The colour of her mucous membranes was poor and she was beginning to run a high temperature. As she collapsed onto the straw, her normally bright eyes were dull, as though she had lost hope.

My first task was to give her some pain relief and to try and stop her becoming even more toxic than she already was. This accomplished, I rolled up my sleeves and got down in the straw with her to begin the greater challenge of removing the dead foal. I used litres of lubricant to cover the rather dry fetus and luckily at that moment—it was well and truly dark by now —we heard the sound of the horsebox returning from the show. Though surprised, Lynne was quick to grasp what was going on and with her assistance we repelled the foal sufficiently to bring the hind legs out and deliver the little dead colt.

Tilly made no effort to get up. She lay there motionless apart from her breathing, undernourished, very weak and very sick. I gave her everything I could think of that might improve her chances of survival, including several litres of intravenous fluids that I kept in the back of my car for emergencies. I promised to call in the next day, knowing in my heart that her chances were no more than 50-50.

The next morning Lynne got up early, fearing the worst. Welcoming whinnies came from the other boxes but no sound from Tilly's. Unable to bear to look, Lynne decided to feed the other ponies before investigating further. As she scooped the feed into the buckets, there was suddenly an impatient and persistent banging from the far side of the stable yard. None of her ponies normally behaved like that. Glancing around she caught a glimpse of little dun ears and then a muzzle eagerly trying to see over the top of the stable door. Hurry up, Tilly wanted her breakfast!

Well, that was not quite the end of the story. Before my second visit, a large and unpleasant-looking man turned up and said he believed his pony was on the property. Lynne explained the mare's ordeal and said the pony was under veterinary care and it would be best not to move her until her treatment was complete. When I heard this later on in the morning, I gave the little mare some long-acting penicillin just in case she was whisked away. Fortunately her temperature was normal and she was now expected to make an uneventful recovery. Two hours later three large men arrived in a Ford transit van that screeched to an abrupt halt outside the stable. Without a word they lifted the pony through the open back doors and with more squealing of tyres drove away.

That was the last we saw of Tilly. However, she did survive. She was seen grazing the grass verges on a short chain tether a few months later. Such is the unfair lottery of life for both animals and people. At least she had 48 hours of good food, love and care when it was most needed.

8

AN ABOUT TURN

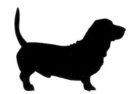

Some days just don't go well. I walked into the office and glanced down the list of visits in the day book. There was only one that I did not particularly want to do; it was to put an elderly basset hound to sleep. Certain breeds of dog, including dachshunds and basset hounds, are notorious for having short and rather twisted legs that can make finding a vein more difficult than in the average dog. With any euthanasia you do everything to make it as calm and peaceful an event as possible for both the pet and its owner, so performing this important task can be quite daunting for a new graduate as there is always the potential for something to go wrong.

My heart sank as Tim picked up his pen and put the letter 'S' (for Sue) beside this particular visit. I had never met the owner or the dog and I did not know the area where they lived. I felt reassured as it was common practice for the vets to take a nurse out with them to hold the animal correctly and raise the vein ready for the injection. But the feeling did not last. Tim was in a grumpy mood and told me that the nurses were too busy so I would have to go on my own.

I drove out to Sturminster Marshall and found the house on the other side of the busy main road. There was nowhere to park so I pulled over into the gateway of a field and made a dash across the road between the continuous streams of traffic. Everything I needed was ready in a stainless steel dish: scissors to clip away the hair, cotton wool and surgical spirit to swab the skin and the injection itself. Instead of a nurse's help, I had a thick elastic band to wrap around the leg to bring up the vein and a pair of artery forceps to hold it in place. With a deep breath, I knocked on the door and waited.

Before the door was halfway open, the verbal assault began.

'I'd like you to know that last time I had a dog put to sleep, it was a complete disaster,' the lady said, glaring at me. 'So I hope you're going to do it well this time.' Then, 'You look a bit young for this job,' she muttered under her breath, turning away. Not a good start. Whilst quivering inside I assured her as confidently as I could that I would do everything possible to make sure that her dog went peacefully. I followed her into the kitchen and put the dish on the table, but there was no sign of the dog.

'Where is he?' I asked, keen to get this task completed.

She pointed to a dark shape on the carpet in the adjoining dining area. The light was poor so I took a step towards the prone dog but stopped in my tracks as he lifted his lip and emitted a blood-curdling growl. I ventured a step closer and as my eyes became accustomed to the dim light, I realised that the poor fellow was in circulatory failure. He was vastly overweight and his distended abdomen spread across the floor. There was no shape to his puffy, oedematous legs and that meant the chances of successfully finding a vein at the first attempt were significantly reduced; that is, if I could get close enough to attempt it. For the next few minutes, I spoke gently to the dog, trying to gain his trust, but he was having none of it. With the lady still complaining and the dog unapproachable, I decided this was mission impossible.

At that moment I could see only one solution. We had no mobile phones in those days but I would go out to the car and use the radio to say that I needed to come back and collect a nurse to help me. Unfortunately Tim was in reception and on hearing my request, he proceeded to give me a lecture on how this should all be within my capabilities by now. With a sinking heart, I realised that I would have to somehow muzzle the dog and inject him with some sedative to make him quiet enough for me to do the deed. Feeling a mixture of irritation with Tim and anxiety about the whole situation, I opened the back door of the car to reach for the case where I kept the powerful sedatives.

At that moment a flash of movement registered in the corner of my eye and I realised to my horror that Poppy, my tricolour Cavalier King Charles puppy, had leapt out of the car and was now on the opposite side of the carriageway in the path of a rapidly approaching lorry. I screamed her name in panic and the little dog froze as the juggernaut passed right over the top of her at 50 miles per hour. Fortunately she was completely unharmed and I was able to scoop her up, dive into the car and give her a cuddle. Trembling and ashen-faced, I crossed the road and went back into the house.

'Whatever is the matter?' asked the lady in genuine concern.

When I explained what had occurred, she became a completely different person.

'Come and sit down whilst I make you a nice cup of tea.' Then she said, 'Don't worry about my dog; he's a grumpy old thing but he'll let you inject the sedative if I hold him. We can drink our tea and have a biscuit whilst he falls asleep.'

And that is exactly what happened. After I had successfully sedated him, she kindly led me to the kitchen table and put the kettle on. Fifteen minutes later I was able to put the dog to sleep without any trouble as she talked to him and stroked his head. Together we carried him out into the garden and carefully placed him in a hole that was already prepared. She insisted on writing me a cheque for the practice there and then and we parted on good terms. Her innate kindness as a human being had only momentarily deserted her as she braced herself for the loss of her pet. She thanked me for a job well done and waved me on my way.

9

ZEUS

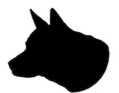

I t was early one Saturday afternoon and I had just finished a few small animal consultations following a morning of large animal visits when a call came in requesting a visit to see a German shepherd dog that was having a fit. He was a very large dog weighing over 40 kilograms and the owners were unable to bring him in as they simply could not lift him. At least, I thought to myself, the address was just around the corner from the practice so I jumped into my car and followed the directions I had been given. Unfortunately they were a bit muddled and after twenty minutes of crawling through the streets, reading the house signs and numbers, I still had not found the house I was looking for.

I called the nurses at the practice on the car radio and asked them to ring the clients on my behalf. This time I arrived safely on the doorstep but the greeting I received was slightly strange. Instead of being hurriedly welcomed and rushed through to my patient, there was an unexplained hesitancy about letting me in. They eventually opened the door and showed me into the lounge but there was no dog to be seen. The owner explained to me that Zeus the dog had now come round and was in the kitchen. Apparently he was a little wary of strangers so 'would I mind taking a seat in the lounge whilst they fetched him?' So I did and what a big mistake that was.

I perched on the edge of the sofa whilst the man's wife and grown-up son went to fetch the dog. The room was about twelve feet wide and as the door opposite me opened, I looked up. Framed in the doorway with two people holding onto his collar was a huge and ferocious-looking dog.

'Sit still and he'll be fine with you,' said the man standing beside me. With that, the dog lurched forwards and pulled free in an instant, springing towards me. 'Don't move, whatever you do,' said the man in panic as the dog came to a halt with his bared teeth just an inch in front of my nose. Its lips were curled back in a threatening snarl, exposing an array of frightening-looking teeth, growling menacingly and panting hot breath into my face. I remained completely immobile, hardly breathing, because even the slightest movement would provoke him to attack. With my hands still by my side, I resisted the urge to cover my face, waiting for the owners to restrain and remove the dog. But no one else moved either. Seconds ticked away, and still nothing. Surely they would rescue me from my predicament. But no.

When I realised that the next step was up to me, I adopted a very calm and low tone in ventriloquist style and said, 'Get the dog out of here,' knowing that if my lips even moved, the dog would tear my face apart.

With that the client grasped the collar and pulled him away. Still not moving and speaking quietly, I instructed them to take the dog out of the room and close the door. Only when it was firmly closed did I stand up and address the people in the room with me, asking how they could possibly invite me into such a situation when they clearly were well aware of the risks. I asked them to make an appointment at the surgery to discuss Zeus's ongoing management (hopefully whilst I was out on my other calls) and they sheepishly agreed. I left the house with a huge sigh of relief. It had been a very narrow escape.

10

NIGHT ATTIRE

A veterinary surgeon's working wardrobe usually contains practical, comfortable and clean clothes—at least at the start of the day. I've learnt over the years not to stray too far from the norm. If you try to pop in and take a quick look at a patient on the way out to somewhere special, that will for sure be the time that the horse wipes his nose or mouth on your top and stains it with mud, snot or green saliva. Equally, when the phone rings just as you are leaving to go to a party, it is best by far to slip back into the work clothes rather than throw overalls or a white coat over the pretty dress. Otherwise you only make the client feel guilty and apologise which is, of course, completely inappropriate and you then spend much longer than normal examining and treating the animal to reassure the client he or she is not spoiling your evening.

However, there is a lesson I learnt the hard way. The owners of a local stable yard were experiencing an unusually high incidence of unexplained colic in their horses. It was my fourth consecutive night on duty and I had been called out in the early hours of the previous three nights. Examining a horse with colic is potentially a messy business as you need to perform a rectal examination and possibly pass a stomach tube. Before starting I always pulled on waterproof trousers and a light waterproof top over my clothes. Each time, the owner's daughters, who were about my age, greeted me wearing dressing gowns and coats over their nighties and pyjamas.

Thus when the call came at 1 a.m. on the fourth night running, I knew what was required and reckoned that no one would notice if I didn't get dressed but put the waterproofs straight on top of my pyjamas before leaving home. That way I could jump straight back into bed afterwards. The girls were waiting anxiously as usual and whilst I examined and treated the horse, we went through all the possible causes of these colics as the laboratory tests done so far had ruled out a number of things but had not been helpful in pinpointing the issue. It was only when I did a postmortem on the worst-affected horse two days later and we found its large intestine full of ingested sand that we knew exactly what the problem was.

After I'd made the horse more comfortable, I was just getting back into my car and preparing to leave when the radio crackled into life and I was instructed to attend a cow that was bleeding badly after calving some distance away. Hmmm, well this was a different situation altogether and I briefly wondered if I could shoot back home and get dressed as I did not feel nearly so comfortable going to a farm call in my pyjamas. The cow's life was in danger and a few minutes could make all the difference so there was no real choice. Half an hour later, with the cow's torn artery successfully clamped, I hosed my waterproofs down and smiled to myself as no one had noticed and I'd got away with it.

I was on my way home when the nurse who had the phones that night got in touch to say there was now an urgent case of milk fever. This is a metabolic disease that occurs at the time of calving or shortly afterwards because the cow's calcium levels become depleted due to the demands of the developing calf and the sudden increase in colostrum and milk production. In the early stages of the disease, the cow trembles and walks stiffly or staggers about, but very quickly she sits down and is unable to get up as her muscles no longer work properly. If left untreated she will progress to lying flat out, often bloated and barely conscious before slipping away towards an uncomfortable death.

It was just beginning to get light at this stage and the first signs of dawn were visible on the horizon. As I drove up to the dairy, I could see the cow was in a bad way, stretched out on the concrete yard. The dairyman had been unable to do much on his own apart from administer some calcium with a large injection under her skin. Between us we worked fast to prop her up with straw bales into a sitting position and relieve the bloat that was making her breathing so laboured. A bottle of calcium borogluconate was warming up to body temperature in a bucket of clean, warm water nearby and as soon as she was in a comfortable position, I administered this directly into a large vein in her neck. As we stood and waited for her to respond, the farmer arrived and asked if I could check another cow that was having difficulty calving in the adjacent yard. Thankfully I was able to deliver the calf without any problem and by that time the cow with milk fever was much brighter. Her head had previously been turned right back so it rested on her flank but now she was sitting upright and alert, taking an interest in her surroundings.

With a glance at my watch, I saw that it was now ten to eight and my small animal surgery started in 40 minutes. Only then did I remember that I was still in my pyjamas and a white coat was not going to hide them from the clients. Confession time— to the nurses at least—who covered for me and explained to the partners that after my busy night I needed to go home to shower and change before starting the morning consultations. Never again have I gone to work without getting dressed properly first.

11

PRINCE

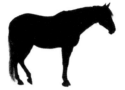

There is no doubt that some horses enjoy a better life than
others. Occasionally my calls would take me to see horses
and ponies that deserved so much more than the bare patch of
earth where they wandered amongst empty tins and broken
glass bottles, fenced in with loose strands of rusty barbed wire.
They often looked depressed, with their heads held low and
their dull eyes glazed over, as though they had mentally
retreated from the barren environment that was their home.
Their owners were not intentionally unkind but simply
misguided, often without the knowledge or funds to provide
proper, basic care for these poor animals. I would willingly
spend time discussing their care, doing what I could to improve
their lives.

Sometimes though a horse's lot is greatly improved by the
kindness and generosity of local people who witness its plight.
One evening I was called to see a horse named Prince. He was a
large and solid gelding, tethered on a piece of grass close to the
edge of a housing estate. He obviously had enough to eat as he
was in good condition and there was shade for him from a
nearby tree, under which was a bucket of fresh, clean water.

Prince was experiencing abdominal pain and I was surprised to learn that the lady who called me out did not own him. She explained that he had lived on this piece of ground for fifteen years and during that time they hardly ever saw his owner, so a group of them clubbed together to provide and care for him.

Prince was sweating lightly and every now and then he tried to lie down. I took his pulse, examined the colour of his membranes and listened to his abdomen with my stethoscope. When I pulled on some long gloves and did an internal examination, my suspicions were confirmed. The poor horse had an impaction of his large bowel and would need assistance to get his gut working normally again. Whilst I was examining him, the sun had set and darkness began to settle. When I looked up, I was surprised to see that a crowd of 20-30 people had gathered around and were quietly waiting in hushed silence to learn Prince's fate. There was an audible sigh of relief when I explained that with treatment he should be absolutely fine.

There was no shortage of volunteers to provide me with buckets of warm water as I made up a mixture with liquid paraffin to stimulate his gut to work and lubricate the dry contents so he could hopefully pass them more easily. After he'd received some fast-acting pain relief intravenously, the trusting horse stood quietly as I passed the warmed stomach tube up his left nostril and he obligingly swallowed at the right moment so the tube passed into his gullet. I then attached a funnel to the tube and steadily poured the warm liquid paraffin mixture into his stomach. By now I could hear some encouraging gut sounds without needing the stethoscope and I gratefully accepted the mug of tea that someone placed in my hand. We stood quietly in the dark and monitored the horse for the next half hour. Thankfully he seemed much more comfortable. A rota of local householders was organised to keep an eye on him throughout the night and I left my phone number in case they had any worries.

At 11p.m. I had a call to say that he seemed back to normal, so I went to bed happy. The next morning I called in and was delighted to find he had passed several piles of droppings, some of which were glistening with liquid paraffin. We also wormed him and later in the week I popped by to rasp his teeth to make sure he could chew his food properly. I learnt that he was a favourite with the local children who had been known to release him from his tether and take him for walks. The gentle giant never took advantage and plodded happily along beside them, enjoying all the attention and the freedom to stretch his legs. It had been a memorable evening with a horse that was loved and cared for by many people and I felt privileged to have played my small part.

12

SHOT IN THE EYE

'I need a vet out right now. My cow has been shot in the eye,' said the voice down the phone.

Oh my goodness, how on earth do I tackle that? I thought to myself. Worse still, this particular farmer was not one of my favourites. He'd made it perfectly clear on my previous visits that I was still very much on trial and for sure he would be watching my every move. Typically it was early on a Saturday afternoon so I was now on duty for the weekend without anyone available to confer with at the surgery. I followed one of the two golden rules suggested by Jim Pinsent, our wonderful large animal lecturer at Bristol Vet School. Jim was an amazing clinician and a kind, patient tutor. When he described a sick animal, his words conjured up an image of the cow or horse so clearly that it could have been with us in the classroom. 'Hurry slowly,' were his words of wisdom when confronted with an unusual or difficult situation, allowing you to drive safely and have a few moments of thinking time, rather than arriving in a compete flap.

By the time I arrived just fifteen minutes later, I could see that the cow was a young heifer and she was standing quietly in the cattle crush. She did not appear to be in great distress, unlike the farmer who was looking pointedly at his watch and champing at the bit. I jumped out of the car, already attired in green overalls, and walked briskly up to the crush with an air of purpose and bid him good afternoon. My greeting was not returned as stony-faced he nodded at the heifer, whose head was helpfully clamped by the crush.

One eye was half closed with tears running down her cheek. There was a distinctive circular white lesion on the clear cornea at the front of the eye and I inwardly heaved a sigh of relief. This was not a wound from a shotgun pellet but an advanced case of New Forest Eye, a disease caused by bacteria and spread from animal to animal by flies and dust. It begins as conjunctivitis and can progress to ulceration of the cornea and even blindness if not treated early enough. It is extremely painful and debilitating so I could see why the farmer had jumped to the conclusion that she had been shot. I decided to explain this tactfully so the farmer would not feel uncomfortable.

I'd barely got beyond sharing the good news that no one was taking pot shots at his cows when he raised himself to his full height of over six foot and said, 'Young lady, you have absolutely no idea what you're talking about.'

I'd noticed the rest of the group of young heifers on the other side of the yard, so I suggested that we strolled over and had a look at them. Sure enough at least half of them were also developing the condition and required treatment. It transpired that they had just been brought up from the meadows and had not been closely observed for a week. I explained that if we treated the young cattle that had runny eyes with some ointment for a few days, this would prevent them progressing to the more serious ulcerative stage. Those with ulcers, however, would need injections of antibiotic under the conjunctiva.

As we walked back to the heifer in the cattle crush, the

farmer was still grumbling about my inability to diagnose what was clearly a gunshot wound.

'Well not to worry,' I said, 'We can agree to differ on the cause of the problem but luckily the treatment is the same.' I collected a bottle of oxytetracycline from the car and drew a small amount into a 2 ml syringe. For a moment I was perplexed as the normally pale golden-brown liquid looked very dark—in fact almost black. Not sure why this was the case (I later learnt that this often happens once the bottle is opened), I decided not to take any chances as I was going to inject it into such a delicate area so I returned to the boot of my car to fetch another bottle. Luckily I always had a spare of the most commonly used treatments.

The grumbling continued and now included comments about my incompetence to even choose the right medication. I was clearly not going to win the farmer over that day so I asked him to hold the animal's head firmly whilst I carefully injected the antibiotic beneath the conjunctiva of her badly infected eye. With that task safely accomplished, we let her loose and ran the rest of the group through the crush so their eyes could be checked and treated as necessary.

An hour later I washed my hands and hosed the muck off my boots, feeling happy that I had done a good job. Although I would have liked to follow this case up myself, I knew the farmer would not be happy so I suggested that one of the other vets should check her in a couple of days during his routine weekly visit. When I looked around to say goodbye, there was no sign of the man. He had already gone without so much as a word of thanks.

I am pleased to say that the story had a happy ending. In the months that followed, I attended several emergencies at the farmer's dairies including calvings, collapsed and injured cows, mastitis and milk fever cases, with mostly successful outcomes. I was always thankful that the farmer was not around and I could get on and work with the dairymen who were invariably friendly. Then one day I saw the farmer at a petrol station and quickly looked the other way, hoping not to catch his eye. He came over with a smile and thanked me for my 'new' way of approaching various problems and said one of his dairymen had been particularly impressed with the way I had dealt with a cow that had done the splits on the concrete. He said I was welcome on any of his farms and invited me for a tour of the estate. Phew! It had taken time to gain his trust but the encounter left me feeling pleased that I now had another satisfied customer.

13

THE ARRIVAL OF HONEY

By now I was happily settled into the routine—or rather the lack of it—of mixed veterinary practice. Work was exciting, challenging and sometimes scary, but never dull. I had a really nice group of friends, my horse to ride and two growing-up puppies. What more could I want?

I will never forget the morning when Mrs Bird came into the surgery and put her six-month golden retriever onto the consulting room table. As I looked at Honey, my heart just melted and I couldn't help saying, 'Oh you are lucky. I dream of owning a dog like this.'

'Well you can have her if you like,' came the reply. I listened in stunned silence as she explained that she had bought two pups—a bitch and a dog—and between them they were destroying her house. And now the dog was bullying Honey so one of them had to be re-homed.

Two things stopped me saying yes there and then. Firstly, I was about to spend a few days in Jersey as my father was very poorly. Secondly, I was now engaged to John, who I'd met during my first summer in Corfe Mullen, so perhaps he should be involved in the decision too. We had recently moved from my

46

rented house and had no restrictions on keeping a large dog so there was no problem there. It was easily solved. Mrs Bird was happy to keep her for a little longer and I would give Honey to John as a present so he would find it difficult to say no. With typical good humour, John gave me a quizzical look when I told him to shut his eyes and then brought Honey in from the car. It was the beginning of fifteen very happy golden retriever years.

A few things changed as a result. Three dogs now occupied the back seat of my car and all of them loved coming to work with me. Most days I passed through the New Forest and was able to take them for a run and as they were well behaved, my clients often invited them out to play. There were some embarrassing incidents when I arrived back at the practice and could not find the day's milk and dung samples destined for the laboratory. A few chewed-up bits of plastic were the clue to their mysterious disappearance and I had to re-visit a number of farmers and explain that their samples were now inside the golden retriever. Thankfully she did not come to any harm as a result.

Then one night I had a bit of a shock whilst watching the 6 o'clock news. It was one of those rare evenings when I was not on duty and had arrived home in time to catch the headlines. I sat bolt upright when the newsreader announced that a police surgeon and a veterinary surgeon had been called in to identify the likely origin of some testicles that had been found by the roadside in St Leonards, Dorset. I felt my face go red and my heart began to beat faster as I thought, *Surely not?* I cast my mind back to earlier in the day when I had castrated an Arab colt close to this location. It was a beautiful sunny morning and the procedure had been very straightforward. As I put the removed testicles in the boot of my car, I realised that if I was not careful, they were likely to become another tasty treat for Honey so I asked the owner of the horse if he would be kind enough to dispose of them for me. But now I could not help wondering... Should I ring him? But then I decided that as they had been identified as horse testicles, perhaps for the moment I should let sleeping dogs lie.

The next time I visited the client, I casually enquired what he had done with the testicles. 'Well, I put them in the passenger footwell of my car but when my wife got in she said they made her feel sick so I lobbed them out of the window,' was his response. I learnt my lesson and that was the last time I asked a client to dispose of my clinical waste. I purchased a dog-proof plastic box with a firmly sealed lid for all those choice treats that were otherwise so very tempting.

14

STUCK IN THE BOG

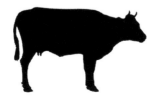

It was very early one morning when I was asked to go to Willow Farm. One of the cows was stuck in a bog and the firemen had asked for a vet to be present as they tried to rescue her. I checked that my long, thick rope was in the boot of my car and set off, confident that I would be able to help. In the early dawn light, the fireman's powerful torches lit up the scene and I drove across the field and pulled up beside the two red fire engines. Everyone was so focussed on the cow that they did not notice my arrival. I made my way over to Mr Birch, the farmer, to let him know that I was there and ready if they needed my help.

The firemen were making heroic efforts to lift the cow out. Two of them had jumped into the thick, black mud and had slid a couple of wide hoses underneath her. But every time they pulled, she came out a little way and then slid backwards into the mire. Feeling shy and rather small beside the hulky firemen, I watched in silence, feeling sorry for the cow that trembling with cold and shock. After a couple more attempts, I tentatively said, 'Excuse me. I know a way to get her out.' Whether they did not hear me or ignored me, I was unsure, but no one paid any attention. I went up to the chap who appeared to be in charge and once again offered my assistance.

'Don't you worry, love. We'll have her out before long,' he said dismissively.

Now beginning to feel a little frustrated at the situation, I went across to Mr Birch and explained that I knew a way to rope her so she could be lifted out and would not slip.

Five minutes later Mr Birch cleared his throat and declared, 'Right chaps, it's Sue's turn now.'

There was a collective raising of eyebrows and murmurs of impatience. In my waders, I grasped the rope and prepared to slide down beside the cow.

'Hang on a moment. If you just give us instructions, we'll do it for you,' exclaimed their chief.

I handed over my long rope and instructed him to make a loop around the cow's neck with the middle of the rope and secure it with a reef knot that would not tighten. Then each of the free ends was passed between the cow's front legs, one behind each elbow and then brought up and crossed over the middle of her back. The ends were now passed between the hind legs, one on either side of the udder, and brought up and twisted together beside the head of her tail then passed under the cross on her back, through the neck loop and finally tied with a loop at the cross. With the cow now tied up like a parcel, she could be pulled up without slipping back.

There was a lot of sniggering from the macho chaps and I carried on, trying to ignore their pointed comments about grandmother's knitting. With the rope secured to my satisfaction, they attached the winch to the loop on the cow's back and began to pull. At first she tipped one way and then the other and my heart was in my mouth as she was gradually freed from the thick, clingy mud.

'It will never hold,' they laughed.

Then slowly but surely with the ropes holding the cow

securely and comfortably, they lifted her onto firm ground. From that moment I concentrated on checking her over, getting her warmed up and treating her for shock. Mr Birch came over and thanked me, but there was silence from the rest of the crew as they packed all their gear away.

Just as I was preparing to leave, the fire chief sidled up to my car and cleared his throat. 'Um, I don't suppose you could show us again sometime could you?' Delighted to share yet another of Jim Pinsent's valuable nuggets of information, I drew him a diagram and later that week posted to him a toy cow all tied up with kitchen string as a reminder of our work. Ultimately, it was a joint effort and I could not have managed without the co-operation of our wonderful fire service.

15

SECRET OPS

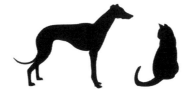

In my second year in Wimborne, one of my university vet friends came to work as a summer locum. She was keen to be involved in farm work but this was mainly a small animal post. I thought there was a good chance that with a little persuasion her role might be extended and so it was that Pippa became my lodger. It was not long before her wish became reality and she was happily included in the large animal duties. She was not so keen on horses, so at the weekends, regardless of who was on duty, I took all the equine emergencies and Pippa attended to the cows.

But we had a secret! I am not sure how it came about but every so often we spent our lunchtime in the operating theatre with a collection of waifs and strays. Such animals were regularly brought into the surgery by the general public and thankfully we had a very good relationship with our local RSPCA inspector who would come and collect them for rehoming. But what about the injured ones? That was a different story and of course the practice could not afford to perform major surgery on every animal with no owner.

The problem was that they were given appropriate first aid

and pain relief for a couple of days to see if anyone came to claim them, but after that...

It all started with a small tortoiseshell cat. She was the sweetest and friendliest of creatures who constantly demanded cuddles and attention despite her very serious injuries. The poor little thing had been caught in some farm machinery whilst it was operating and one eye and a hind leg were beyond repair. The farmer had kindly brought her in but she did not belong to him. What could we do? We asked our friendly RSPCA colleague for a donation to cover the cost of the drugs so the practice would not lose out. That done, we had to enlist the help of the nurses (ie. encourage them to turn a blind eye) and choose our time carefully. On Fridays the partners always went home for lunch and one of them would have the afternoon off, so that lunchtime seemed a good choice.

At 12:30 p.m. we both arrived at the practice just in time to see the partners drive off. Action stations! On with the green operating gowns and for the next hour we did not stop. We gently lifted the little cat, who we unimaginatively named Hoppity One-Eye, onto the operating table and I anaesthetised her so Pippa could perform the surgery. The next patient was a greyhound who had clearly been walking alone in the countryside for a quite a while. He was very thin and the skin on his paws was quite raw. His face was covered in ticks and unfortunately his tail was severely damaged and required partial amputation. So many greyhounds are abandoned once their racing days are over but this patient and gentle dog loved our attention despite his circumstances.

With the surgery done, how did we explain it to the partners? No problem because whenever we had a shy or stressed patient, we would hang a blanket over the front of the kennel to give them some privacy. Who was going to look behind the blanket on a Friday afternoon? Our nurses were particularly good at finding temporary homes for our recovering patients before they began life with a new owner. The greyhound went on to enjoy life with a family on a farm and Hoppity One-Eye lived out her days with an old lady who adored and spoiled her.

The occasional operating days continued for quite a while until Richard strode back into the practice and straight into the operating theatre one Friday afternoon.

'All of these animals are to be gone by Monday and after that, no more please.' He had known for months what was going on and had kindly turned a blind eye, but enough was enough.

16

ROUGH JUSTICE

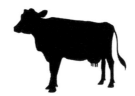

We all know that sometimes life is just not fair. I was reminded of this in my second year of practice after being called to a farm to help a cow that had been unable to deliver a dead calf. Many farmers in the New Forest have grazing rights and their cattle run free so they do not get the same level of supervision as the cows in a dairy herd, who are checked several times a day. This cow had been discovered sitting down, unable to rise, with a calf that had been dead for some time half in and half out of her. He had become stuck at the hips, which had prevented his safe delivery, and without any assistance he had died. Unfortunately the small body had begun to decompose and was now partly missing, probably mauled by a fox in the time that passed before the cow's plight was discovered.

The cow was in a poor way but as she was bright-eyed and sitting up, we decided to give her a chance, since the alternative was euthanasia. The first step was to administer some antibiotics and fluids before tackling the problem at her rear end. Using several bottles of lubricant, I then knelt down and gradually eased my hand inside the cow and established that there was no way the calf's hips would pass through her pelvis. I would have to perform an embryotomy and divide its body into smaller pieces that could be more easily removed. As I lay on the ground, stretching at full reach inside her and my face close to the remains of the calf, I noticed some maggots wriggling in my peripheral vision.

With some difficulty, as the uterus was tightly clamped around the hips, I managed to position the embryotomy wire between the calf's back legs with the two free ends outside the cow. Standing up, I aligned the wires so they would not damage the cow and began to saw through the calf's pelvis. It was hard work but I had got into the swing of it when the farmer asked if he should take over. I hesitated for a second as everything was coming on nicely, but then thought, *Why not?* and let him step in.

A minute or so later, the job was complete and with care, I was able to remove the remains of the calf in two pieces. We gave the cow some additional drugs to make her more comfortable and reduce the inevitable swelling. Her outlook was still guarded but I was happy that the embryotomy had gone well and she did not seem any the worse after it. With a thank you and cheery goodbye from the farmer, I left to continue with my other calls.

The following evening a friend came to supper and said that he had repaired some machinery at the same farm earlier in the day and heard all about the cow's ordeal. Apparently she was looking bright and the farmer was full of praise for my efforts. It gave me a warm glow as I remembered the physical effort involved and the ghastly maggots. I crossed my fingers for a happy outcome.

A fortnight later I was surprised to be called in to see Tim and almost speechless when he read out the letter in his hand. The farmer was refusing to pay the bill as his cow had died and the young vet (me) that attended was apparently so incompetent that he had needed to take over the embryotomy himself. How the tables had turned. Deeply hurt at the injustice and disappointed by the cow's death, I gave Tim an accurate version of events, which he accepted. I never went there again and 35 years on, I still remember that day and feel sad whenever my travels take me past the farm.

A BUSY DAY

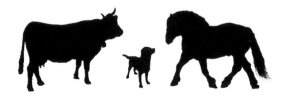

I felt really good as I popped into the office to pick up my list of calls. I'd been in the practice for quite a time now and I had built a good relationship with several clients who would phone up and ask specifically for me when they had a problem. The nurses always wrote the initial of the requested vet in the margin of the page by the visit and between us we would then allocate the remaining visits according to our schedule and geographical route. I much preferred doing the farm and horse calls rather than the small animal consultations or operating list. Today I knew I was guaranteed to be busy until my evening surgery, which started at 6 p.m.

As I looked down the list, I noticed that there was a litter of twelve German shepherd dog puppies needing a second vaccination and the owners lived along the same road as my first colt castrate of the day. I would pass by their door on the way to see the horse but I had so much other work that I really hoped I would not be asked to go there. Our practice policy was to give the puppies a very thorough clinical examination at the time of the first vaccination and issue the certificates with the puppies' details and the batch numbers of the vaccines with the second injection.

In the days before computerised records, I needed to find the record card and write out all the relevant information as I vaccinated each pup and this would take more time than I had available. A glance at the rest of the list showed me that the other vets had much lighter schedules and could easily accommodate this task. In any case the pups belonged to a lovely client who was kind enough to look after my dogs when I went away on holiday, so I did not want to be just dashing in and out.

I copied the list of visits to my diary and looked forward to the day. I had two colts to castrate, a lame horse to examine, an off-colour goat, a pre-purchase examination of a horse, a horse to X-ray and eighteen cows on two separate farms to examine to determine whether they were in calf.

I looked around quickly and was just making my escape through the front door of the practice when I heard the sound of Tim's voice. 'Ahem... Sue.' I debated carrying on and pretending I had not heard but then decided I had better stop and listen to what he had to say. After all, it may have nothing to do with the twelve pups. Alas it did and although I protested quite strongly, he'd made up his mind. In a moment of pure exasperation, I ripped the page out of the day book with a flourish, stating that I might as well take it with me since I was doing all of the work anyway. With that I grabbed the vaccines given to me by a surprised-looking nurse then turned on my heel and left without looking back.

Still feeling cross I decided to go and see the pups first which was a good move as their friendly welcome instantly calmed me down. The clients were old hands at this and between us we vaccinated all twelve and wrote out their certificates in record time. They even placed a mug of tea in my hand as I left to see the colt another mile down the bumpy track and said to drop off the empty mug on my way back.

From then on the day went smoothly enough until I got to the last farm which was on the outskirts of the practice area. The fourteen cows I had expected had somehow become twenty-one and it was now 5 p.m. so I had a decision to make. Was I or was I not going back for my evening surgery? In an instant I decided that someone else would have to stand in for me and I got on with the business of examining all of the cows. The dairyman was not feeling well so it took a little longer than usual but as it was my final visit of the day, we just took our time until we'd accomplished all the tasks.

It was not until I was hosing all the cow dung from my gown and boots that I began to worry that there might be consequences to my morning strop. There was plenty of time to think about it as I drove back across the hills with panoramic views of farmland on either side of the road in the low evening sun. Although I knew I should not have left in such a manner, I still felt I was justified in complaining and was not about to grovel and say sorry, so it was difficult to see how this could be resolved amicably.

Still uncertain I got out of the car and walked into the reception area and looked around enquiringly. Evening surgery had finished and the nurses who were tidying up seemed quietly amused as I sellotaped the page back into the day book and started to fill in the list of drugs that I had used at each visit. Then all of a sudden, the atmosphere in the room changed. The nurses became very busy and I knew without looking that Tim had walked in. I kept my head down and was still writing out my notes when he approached me from behind and with huge aplomb put his arm around my shoulders and smiled, saying, 'Well, Sue, you've had a busy day. Let me make you a cup of tea.' With that, he very cleverly defused the situation humorously with no loss of face to either of us. No more was said and we both went home happy, ready for the next day in the busy mixed practice.

18

A FADING STAR

I t was a chilly November afternoon, already getting dark. I'd popped into the surgery to collect a few drugs when the call came in. Star, a very old pony, had gone down in his stable and Mary, his owner, thought he was dying. Could I please go and look at him straight away and put him out of his misery?

As I jumped into my car, I recalled my visits to see this old pony during the last few months. On each occasion he had a mild grumbling colic that we had tentatively put down to worm damage since many horses and ponies shared the same grazing. He was now 32 years old and had become progressively thinner with time.

There was no sign of any activity when I arrived. The makeshift stables were constructed out of corrugated iron and timbers, but a dim light was visible from the middle stable. Gathering up a few bits of equipment, I quietly opened the door and slipped inside. The moments that followed will stay with me for the rest of my life.

The panic was over; Star lay flat out in the deep straw with Mary gently stroking his head. One glance told me all I needed to know. Apart from very slow, deep breaths, the pony was still.

The brown eyes were unfocused and no help was needed from me. These were the last moments of this pony's life.

I quietly told Mary that Star was not in any pain but dying peacefully and I asked if she would like to be alone or prefer me to stay. I felt very privileged to be invited to share the next few minutes. As I knelt beside the fading pony, I learnt an important lesson—never judge anyone or anything by their appearance. Not on any of my previous visits did I learn of his incredible achievements. All I had seen was a thin, old pony.

Mary started to tell me of some of the highlights of his show jumping career. In my imagination I was transported from the cold, dimly lit stable to the bright lights of Wembley. Year after year he took different children to success that most of us only dream of. Well into his twenties, he had won the Junior Show Jumper of the Year. I felt humbled and honoured to hear these stories at such a poignant moment.

As his breaths became quieter and more erratic, our thoughts returned from the glory of the past to the special moment now. We sat in silence, each paying tribute to the courage and character of the little bay pony before us.

Gently and peacefully the light of this star was extinguished.

19

LUCY

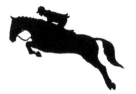

Whilst on the subject of special horses, it was during my years in Wimborne that I finally lost my horse Lucy after ten amazing years together. She was with me throughout my student days and first years in practice. When I had first viewed her, I flew into a small airport in the North of England and was met by a gentleman who spotted me as we had agreed I would be carrying a copy of *Horse & Hound*. That evening we went to an indoor show where I watched his young daughter jump Lucy successfully into fourth place in quite a big class. She was bright bay, ¾ Thoroughbred and stood at just fifteen hands but had huge ability and enthusiasm for the job. The next morning when it was my turn to ride her, I was jumped right out of the saddle but after that we never looked back.

There followed ten years of complete and mutual trust, whether it was taking me round my first-ever cross-country course, jumping a huge fence or hacking through heavy traffic without batting an eyelid. Nothing fazed Lucy. I had little opportunity and no money for any professional training but at the time it did not seem to matter as we tackled everything together with enthusiasm and joy.

Of course there were some magic moments that I will never forget. In my first cross-country competition there was a fence with several telegraph poles one after another at various angles so I had to plan the route and work out the distances to get the striding right. I will never forget the feeling of Lucy lowering her neck to have a good look, pricking her ears and just taking me through.

She was so brave cross country that we were quickly out of novice classes and had to tackle the much bigger, open class fences. There were huge spreads and ditches, water jumps and drops but she never refused and had many wins to her credit. At the beginning of each season, I would walk the course and wonder if my horse really wanted to jump these huge fences— and she always did. But my biggest love was show jumping and still without any training or lessons, she took me round affiliated classes up to grades B and C and won numerous unaffiliated opens.

One of the most memorable moments was a Christmas show jumping meeting at Badgeworth arena when I was still a vet student. By this stage, Lucy was only eligible for open classes. To my disappointment I discovered that if I wanted to jump a second class that day, it would have to be a puissance, a high-jump competition over a reduced number of fences. Not my idea of fun, especially on a small horse, but I entered, deciding that I could always withdraw at the appropriate moment when I felt I'd asked enough of her.

There were around twenty starters—horses and ponies of various shapes and sizes—but quite soon the fences went over 1 m 30 cm and the field was whittled down to half a dozen. It was quite cold and getting dark when a very well-dressed and rather unpleasant man on a huge and smart horse came to stand beside me. He looked down his nose at my little unclipped Thoroughbred mare with rubs on her shoulders from the ghastly, green canvas New Zealand rugs that were the only ones available in those days, and in a patronising voice said, 'You wouldn't think that an animal like that could possibly have any chance in this class.' Well, that was mean.

The competition continued and gradually the other horses were eliminated and soon it was just him and me left. By now the spread fence and the wall were at least 1 m 45 cm and with her usual enthusiasm and pricked ears, Lucy did not hesitate and sailed over. So up went the fences for what I decided would definitely be our last round. This time I took the little white brick off the top of the wall and the other horse knocked a pole down from the huge and wide spread fence. The judge asked if we would like to jump again or share first prize and I quickly offered to share.

'No, she will jump again,' said a voice from behind me and there was my fellow vet student and great friend Sarah, with a huge grin on her face. So once more into the ring and this time I knew I just had to jump clear to win as the other horse went first and had a pole down. As usual Lucy took charge and arrived at the huge spread fence on a perfect stride, giving a wonderful sensation of power as she cleared it easily. So now it was just the wall and my heart was in my mouth as we approached it for the last time.

I was so proud when Lucy skimmed over the top and won the class. My little horse who lived out all year round had put the unkind man in his place. The bonus was that the prize was a large Christmas turkey and since it did not fit in our fridge and we had no freezer, it provided a very special, end-of-term meal for half a dozen hungry vet students. I was touched when just as we were about to start eating, one of my friends proposed a toast: 'To Lucy.'

She was definitely my horse of a lifetime. I was pleased that I could give her the stable and luxuries she deserved during her last years. And when she had gone, I discovered that actually I now had to learn to ride, which was humbling and a challenge I am still trying to achieve.

20

CHANGES ON THE HORIZON

By the summer of 1986, I was beginning to get itchy feet. I loved my job in mixed practice and thanks to my wonderful colleagues and the opportunities that had come my way, I now felt competent at tackling most challenges. The three years had passed with a non-stop succession of late-night and early-morning farm calls and a huge variety of animals to treat. But in my heart, I dreamt of being a horse vet and was ready to move on. I went for an interview at a large mixed practice in Salisbury and was delighted to be offered a job as an equine assistant. But they wanted me to start in four weeks, which was less than my notice period in Wimborne. Feeling burdened with this choice, I went to Richard's house and broke the news. To his absolute credit, he gave me a hug and wished me good luck. Being older and wiser he had seen this coming so it was no surprise. With a parting gift of a gold carriage clock, which still sits on my mantelpiece today, I packed my bags and headed for Salisbury.

That summer I changed jobs, moved house and got married to John. Jayne and my sister Jane were my bridesmaids, looking stunning in deep rust-red dresses on an early September day, complemented by my four-year-old niece Kerry in ivory that matched my own dress with a rust-coloured sash around her waist.

Sadly my father had died of leukaemia two years earlier so I walked down the aisle of Canford Church on the vicar's arm. It gave me huge comfort that Dad had lived to see me happily working as a country vet. Years earlier when I was studying at Oxford University, I had approached him on a sunny day when he was working in his beloved garden. 'Hey, Dad. If I could get a place at vet school by any chance, would you please consider supporting me until a time when I could repay you?' He put down his fork and told me that if I had asked to do anything else, the answer would be no. But in his opinion I was born to care for animals so I could apply to vet school and he shared my delight when I was accepted at Bristol University.

In my first summer in practice, he knew the end was near and I was summoned for 'a quiet word' as he wanted to know my plans. He told me to look at my two younger sisters who had good jobs (pharmacist and nurse), husbands and homes. And what did I have? Two puppies, a much-loved horse and an empty bank account with little prospect of owning a house. He wanted to make sure that I was going to be OK. I remember that moment in my kitchen when I was able to smile and tell him that he had given me the greatest gift and opportunity possible. I was now living my dream and wanted for nothing.

John and I rented a semi-detached cottage on the top of the hill at Odstock with the estate shepherd as our only neighbour for miles around. Thankfully it was summer as there was no heating and apart from the kitchen, each room had only a single power point for an old-fashioned, round-pin plug. We still had very few material possessions. Lucy had come to the end of her days but Twiggy, Poppy and now William, the Cavalier King Charles spaniels, and Honey the golden retriever settled delightedly into their new country home.

It was certainly all change at work as I went from being the popular horse vet to the new one that no one wanted. On my very first day, I had sorted out the practice car and filled the boot with all the drugs and equipment I thought I might need. Now back in the vets' office, I looked longingly at the visit book with the list of calls for each vet. All of the clients had requested a particular vet so I was there to await any emergencies. I did not mind as I enjoyed that aspect of the work but I was keen to get started. At that moment one of the secretaries came in and asked, 'Have you seen any of the farm vets? There's a difficult calving to do at West Dean and I think all four of the farm vets are tied up or some distance away.'

'Well, I can do it,' I offered.

'You? But you're a horse vet,' came the reply.

'Ah, but I was a farm vet last week,' I answered.

Looking a bit nonplussed, she telephoned David, one of the senior farm vets and asked if that would be OK. He said to go ahead so I popped down to the dispensary and looked around for any equipment I might need. To my delight there was a spare calving aid propped against the wall so I grabbed it, together with some cow pessaries and some extra calving ropes, and set off.

The farmer was definitely surprised to see me but we quickly got on with the task. I reached inside the cow and discovered that the calf was presented all wrong. All I could feel at first were two front feet but no head. As I extended my arm further, I found that its head was turned backwards over its shoulder and was at the limit of my reach. It was going to be challenging but I was reasonably certain that with a bit of patience I would be able to bring the head round and deliver the calf.

Shortly after that, David arrived to see how I was getting on. In his friendly manner, he said he could stay and help or continue with his already busy day. Crossing my fingers I told him to carry on with his calls, keen to do something useful on my first day. Now I was going to have to get the calf out successfully. Shortly afterwards I managed to put a rope over the calf's jaw and slowly turned its head into the correct position for delivery. With the aid of a whole bottle of gel lubricant, I manoeuvred the calf and with the assistance of a few helpful pushes from the cow, who had been remarkably stoical and stood completely still whilst this was going on, the calf emerged. We held it upside down for a moment to help clear its airways and then settled it on the straw and gave its chest a good rub. With that the little creature shook its head and began to breathe normally.

I hosed myself down, scrubbed my boots and cleaned the equipment before putting it back in the car. As I drove back to the practice, I had a good feeling, happy to have been useful, even if my first job as a dedicated horse vet was to deliver a calf.

It did not take long for me to become busy in my own right. A few of my Wimborne clients tracked me down and I quickly made friends and gained the respect of new clients. I worked incredibly hard and learnt new skills with ups and downs along the way.

As winter settled in and even the water in our loo froze overnight, John and I decided that it was time to make more effort to find a house of our own. On one occasion we were gazumped at the last minute but then on New Year's Eve we spotted a house in an estate agent's window that seemed to be everything we were looking for. We drove by it the next day and as I looked over the gate at the pretty, late-Victorian cottage with its lawns, shrubs, silver birch trees and attached paddock, I was filled with the certain knowledge that I would be very happy there. The negotiations were long and tricky, not to mention nerve-racking, but in February 1987 we moved into the village of Farley, which has been my home ever since.

21

NIGHT ADVENTURE

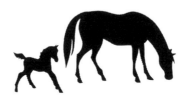

One of my favourite new clients was a lady called Sue. When the out-of-hours telephone lady called one night to say that Sue needed to speak to me urgently, I wasn't sure whether to smile to myself or wait with trepidation to find out what sort of escapade we were going on this time.

I didn't have to wait long before finding out. 'There's a little mare in the graveyard at Woodgreen,' explained Sue, 'and the afterbirth has been hanging from her for at least 24 hours now.' Such cases were never without a variety of complications quite apart from catching and handling a wild pony in the New Forest. For a start, who did it belong to? Would they consent to the treatment and were they going to pay?

Luckily Sue was well acquainted with these dilemmas and had established that the owner didn't mind what we did provided he didn't receive a bill. His feelings were that she could take her chance along with the other foaling mares. Poor Sue, who'd seen the pony, was too concerned to leave her. One of the worst complications of having a retained afterbirth in the pony is a serious and toxic laminitis causing excruciating foot pain, which even with prompt treatment can end in the death of the unfortunate animal.

The mare was grey but she was so muddy, it was difficult to tell in the pitch black. I was given directions to an old church deep in the forest, far from any sign of civilisation. It was bitingly cold as I crawled slowly along the frozen tracks with my headlights on full beam, trying to locate Sue and the pony. Thankfully after what seemed like miles of dead bracken and bare, shrubby bushes, I spied the familiar green Morris Minor with the back doors open. Quite unperturbed, the pony was munching the bale of hay in the boot and Sue was quietly talking to her to gain her confidence.

It never ceases to amaze me just how much you can do to an untamed pony. They truly seem to sense that you are acting for their benefit and their trust is a feeling which grows within minutes as you proceed with whatever job has to be done. Sure enough the ragged and now filthy placenta was trailing behind the little mare. Since the terrain was rather hazardous with overgrown and fallen gravestones hidden beneath the undergrowth, we decided that our first task was to anchor the patient. We gently slipped on the rope halter that I keep in my car for these occasions and apart from one brief, wary look from the pony, the munching sound remained uninterrupted as I tightened the rope. In fact the mare was so intent on the unexpected feast that she virtually ignored the timid little foal that remained half hidden in the bushes.

After I'd put on a pair of disposable, arm-length gloves, I slowly twisted up and applied gentle traction to the placenta, which showed no signs of detaching. There was nothing for it but to try and give the mare a drug to separate and expel it. The only problem was that it needed to be given slowly over several minutes. Well, nothing ventured, nothing gained, so why not?

Whilst Sue fed her some even more delicious carrots and held the torch, I clipped a patch of hair from over the pony's jugular vein, put a small amount of local anaesthetic under the skin and slid a catheter directly into her bloodstream. Within seconds I'd attached a drip tube and bag containing the vital drug. All we had to do was to keep our patient interested enough to stay around. At about this point, we began to laugh at the odd situation—here we were with a wild pony attached to a drip in the middle of a pitch-black graveyard.

Thankfully the placenta dropped away a while later and for good measure we infused some antibiotics as well. The foal was suckling his mum as we quietly drove away. Yet another happy patient, especially as we left her some hay. All in all a very satisfying and worthwhile night's work.

22

OFF WITH HIS...

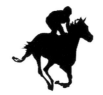

I know several racehorse trainers and almost without exception they are charming people. Not only do they use their knowledge and skill to train the young horses but they also entertain the owners with great bonhomie both at home and on the racecourse. However, there is always the odd one out and I came across a particular individual who had no time for women vets and no qualms about letting them know how he felt. Naturally I did not enjoy working for the man, whom I considered to be brusque and rude, so when I was diverted from my routine calls to go to the gallops and attend to a horse with a broken leg, I was on full alert on several counts. The message had come in that the horse's leg was swinging in the breeze, which suggested this was a catastrophic injury from which the horse could not recover.

My primary concern was to get there as soon as possible to assess the situation and either stabilize the fracture and provide some pain relief or else put the poor creature out of its misery. It also went through my mind that the trainer would be upset and I therefore braced myself not only for the unpleasant deed but the likelihood that he would be even more terse than usual.

To make everything as smooth and efficient as possible, I pulled over briefly as I reached the track up to the gallops and retrieved the gun from a secure hidden compartment in my car, in case I needed it. I put a single bullet into the chamber and with the safety catch on, slid the gun under a copy of *Horse & Hound* so it was hidden from view on the front passenger seat of the car.

It was a grey, windy day and the car bumped from side to side as I picked the best route up the rutted track, concentrating hard and scanning the landscape as I was not familiar with the area and did not know exactly where to find the stricken horse. It came as a complete shock when the passenger door suddenly opened whilst I was still on the move and a large man jumped in and gesticulated that I should go straight ahead. He seemed to materialise from nowhere but must have been hidden from view by the hedge.

As he gave me directions, two thoughts went through my mind. Firstly, I was not entirely sure who this man was as the trainer had never previously bothered to speak to me and I had only seen him at some distance, and secondly, whoever he may be, he was now sitting on top of the loaded gun. Although it was not cocked and therefore could not go off, I was very uncomfortable with this inadvertent breach of firearm safety which did not help an already stressful situation. In my mind's eye, I could see tomorrow's newspaper headlines: 'Vet accidentally shoots racehorse trainer!' or 'Vet gets her revenge' and wondered what the Veterinary Defence Society would have to say about that.

As we went over the rise of the hill, it was immediately obvious that this was indeed a disaster. A lad was holding the horse and the lower half of one of the animal's hind limbs was hanging limply at completely the wrong angle. Despite the severity of the injury, the horse had his head held high and was surveying the scenery with pricked ears. I conveyed my sympathy to the trainer and was thankful that he jumped out of the car without looking back so I could grasp the gun from the seat just vacated by his backside. In such a situation, there is no time for sentiment or to do anything other than examine the horse and then calmly, kindly and safely put an instant and humane end to its pain.

Later on in the day, I learnt that the horse had been considered to have the form and potential to be a star of the future and his death was a huge loss to everyone involved with him. His demise did make headlines on the racing pages of the national papers but thankfully not in the way I had imagined earlier.

23

THE RELUCTANT COLT

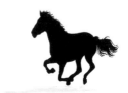

Things don't always go right and some clients seem to set things up so that they consistently go wrong. So it was with Mrs Humphries. I had been to her old, grey stone farmhouse on several occasions, each time to see an unusual case. Today should be quite straightforward as she had a large colt that needed to be castrated. I was pleased to have Tom, a young vet student, with me as Mrs Humphries was quite elderly and unsteady on her limbs. I always enjoyed the company of students and as I gained in experience myself, I was pleased to share with them all the helpful tips I had learnt over the years.

As instructed we called at the house to collect Mrs Humphries on the way to the field. We used the knocker and rang the large, brass bell that hung outside the front door. The blue paint had seen better days and was peeling off in large strips. When we got no reply, we pushed the door open and made our way into the dark hall. It was very gloomy so I warned Tom about the tortoises and rabbits that shared this part of the house as I did not want him to trip up or for the animals to be accidentally trodden on.

'Mrs Humphries,' I called.

'In the kitchen, my dear,' she replied.

Tom and I navigated the various creatures with some difficulty and made our way to the kitchen where she was boiling up some clean water for the operation. Over the years, I learnt not to trust clients I did not know to provide me with clean buckets and warm water for this procedure as all too often they thought that filthy containers covered in bird poo and water from an old barrel would suffice. In my car was a plastic container with several gallons of warm water and a couple of suitable buckets.

'Don't worry, I've brought some with me,' I said and we helped the old lady into her coat and then onto the front seat of my car.

As I was uncertain of exactly where the colt was, she directed me up a long, stony track to the top of a hill. Tom jumped out and opened the gate. As I drove into the field, I briefly wondered where the patient was as there were no horses in sight. Then I heard a whinny and the thunder of hooves as a group of horses galloped into view.

'That's the one, in the lead. I put him out for a last run with the mares this morning,' said Mrs Humphries, pointing to a large, dark-brown colt as he flew past.

My heart sank. Under normal circumstances, you're presented with a clean, calm animal in well-organised conditions. And here we were, in a huge field on the top of a hill with our patient highly aroused in a lather of sweat and not even caught. My emergency halter came to good use again as Tom and I gradually encouraged the huge animal to come towards the offerings of titbits from our pockets. With a sigh of relief, I slipped the headcollar over his ears and patted his huge neck. The colt towered above me with his flanks heaving and steam rising from his body. What, I wondered, was all this activity doing to his blood pressure?

'I need a calm and relaxed patient before the surgical

procedure as all this excitement increases the risk of complications occurring,' I explained to Mrs Humphries. 'I think perhaps we should organise things differently and come back tomorrow.'

'No other day is possible,' she replied. 'I'm afraid I need you to get on and do it now please.'

Tom walked the colt around to cool him off whilst I stood back to make an assessment of his bodyweight. He must be all of 700 kilogrammes. Such a large animal in a state of excitement would normally require a hefty dose of sedation but as he was part Shire horse, I reduced the amount a little as this breed can be particularly sensitive to the drug I was going to use. The last thing I needed was for him to lie down as this was to be a standing castration. As I laid out my instruments on a sterile cloth, I was pleased to see that he was now much calmer. With everything ready, I raised his jugular vein and slowly injected the sedative. Within a very short time, his head hung low and he seemed nicely asleep. This was the moment to inject local anaesthetic into the testicles to make them completely numb. I reached out and before I had a chance to grasp the furthest testicle, *thwack*, a hoof narrowly missed my head and grazed my left arm. So much for the reduced sedative dose. I now topped him up with more.

For a while things went according to plan. I successfully numbed his testicles with local anaesthetic and thoroughly cleaned them with warm water and surgical scrub. After I'd scrubbed my own hands, I made an incision in his skin and pulled gently down on the first testicle so I could place the sterile emasculators around the exposed cord. This instrument cuts the cord and firmly clamps and crushes the associated blood vessels at the same time to prevent any post-operative bleeding.

A few minutes later, I gently undid the emasculators and watched with satisfaction as the crushed end of the cord was gently retracted and disappeared from view back inside the horse. I mentally relaxed as I made the incision to remove the second testicle, thinking I was almost done. But as I exerted gentle traction on the second testicle, the colt pulled it upwards, making it very difficult to grasp. I allowed him a minute to settle and tried again, with the same result.

After a couple more attempts, we stopped to reassess the situation. The colt still seemed very sleepy and he had been given generous doses of local and intravenous analgesia so he should not be experiencing any discomfort. I resolutely tried a few more times, becoming warm with the effort and trying to ignore the complaining and rapidly fatiguing muscles in my forearms. I began to have visions of myself being pulled up inside the horse's abdomen or the horse waking up and running off with me still grasping his remaining testicle.

I decided to redeploy my assistants. Mrs Humphries could hold the headcollar rope and Tom could quickly scrub up to assist me. Thank heavens for strong young vet students. It was still a struggle but with two hands Tom managed to lower the testicle sufficiently for me to clamp the cord. At last! With the job done, we cleared up and gave the old lady post-operative instructions that we knew were unlikely to be followed.

As we drove away and on to our next visit, I explained to Tom that you could never take anything for granted in this job. Although castrating colts is a common and routine operation, there was always the potential for something unexpected to occur. I chuckled to myself as I recounted the tale of the colt that suddenly lost balance and toppled over onto me as I stood holding the clamped emasculators in place. I was surprised to find myself sitting down with him lying across my lap, his back against my chest. He was only a small animal and I was not hurt but neither could I extract myself from underneath him. The owners were unable to shift him as one had a bad back and the other was too elderly to undertake any weight lifting. In the end they undid the laces and removed the chunky leather boots from my feet which were sticking out on the other side of the sleeping colt. I was then able to wriggle out from underneath him and finish the task whilst he continued to snore gently. All in a day's work!

24

MR CHALKE

'Uh-oh,' I thought as I learnt that Mr Chalke required a visit. It was quarter to eight in the morning and I had had a quiet night on duty which was unusual considering we were now well into the stud season. As I looked out through the French windows at the sunlight filtering through the trees, it crossed my mind that an encounter with Mr Chalke was just what I did not need. I had a full list of calls to make, all to regular clients and I was about to start my rounds. As usual I'd been looking forward to my work and now all that had changed.

I cast my mind back to one evening the previous summer. I was still in the office chatting to the other vets when Lindsay, our receptionist, rushed in looking rather flustered.

'Mr Chalke has a yearling with colic and he wants a visit straight away. The only thing is, he doesn't want you,' she said.

'Why not?' I asked, thinking it was odd since he had not even met me.

'He only wants a man,' came the reply.

I instructed Lindsay to politely inform him that the other equine vet on duty was already out on a call some distance away and that I was on my way. Lindsay reappeared and said he wanted me to know that the colt had been sired by a very famous and successful stallion and was worth in excess of 60,000 guineas. I raised my eyebrows because although this made the colt very valuable to him, the treatment options were the same whether it was a prized stallion or a small pony.

As I drove out along the river valley, I felt annoyed. It's always difficult to go to calls knowing that you are not wanted but especially so as I was now experienced at dealing with colic cases. Even more curiously I felt a few faint twinges of anxiety in my tummy. It was a long time since attending a colic case had made me feel nervous and this man had succeeded in making me cross and nervous in one go.

As I arrived on the farm, an oldish man came out to greet me.

'Mr Chalke? Pleased to meet you,' I said, extending my hand.

'Thank you for coming but there's no need. He's better now,' replied the man abruptly.

As I'd driven some twenty miles at speed, I was certainly not leaving without at least examining the horse. Mr Chalke led me inside a barn and there was a chestnut colt, which I had to agree looked a picture of health. Begrudgingly I was allowed to check the animal over. We discussed the causes of spasmodic colic and how to lessen the chances of it recurring before I bid him good evening and left.

Well, back to this particular morning. The telephone lady cleared her throat and began rather nervously to say something.

'Don't worry,' I interrupted. 'I know, he doesn't want a lady vet.'

Determined to keep my cool, I asked her to ring him back and offer him a choice of a visit from me now or the possibility of a male vet being free once the early morning stud visits were finished. I was informed that I could come but that I probably would not be able to manage. Apparently a colt had hurt his mouth on the bolt on the stable door and several teeth were hanging loose.

When I arrived I was led to a loose box with a smart-looking, grey colt playing about with something in his mouth. As I gently pulled back his lips, it was easy to see that he had lost a couple of teeth and the gum had been stripped off the jaw bone, which was exposed and splintered in places. The patient was relatively unperturbed considering the extent of his injuries.

Once the colt was sedated, the stud groom led him to the doorway of the box so we could take advantage of the daylight. I knelt down and after injecting some local anaesthetic began snipping away the dead and damaged tissue and tidying up the splintered bone. Far from being intimidated this time, I was really in my element, knowing that all the pieces would come together nicely and he would be absolutely fine. About ten minutes into the job, Mr Chalke arrived.

'I expect you'll need some help with that, won't you?' he asked.

'No, it will be fine,' I replied, concentrating on the task without looking up. As the footsteps receded, I asked the stud groom (who was very friendly and helpful) whether he treated everyone like this.

'Only women,' was the reply.

Half an hour later, I had removed the loose teeth and managed to find enough gum tissue to draw together over the exposed bone. I used tiny sutures that would not need removing but be absorbed with time to minimise the discomfort to the colt. Injuries to the mouth usually heal very well and I was pleased with the result.

As I packed away my instruments in the boot of the car, Mrs Chalke walked up and said she supposed I would have to admit the horse to our hospital for him to be properly repaired. Highly amused by now, I decided to join in the spirit of the moment. Walking over to the colt that was still sleeping off his sedative, his head hanging low, I called them both over. Gently raising the colt's head and lifting his upper lip, I turned to face them.

'Not a bad job for a woman?'

Looking rather sheepish Mr Chalke began to stutter, 'Well, er no, well actually, um, er it looks fine.'

'That's good then,' I replied. 'Please have it checked when your mares are examined on Thursday.'

With that I said goodbye and jumped in my car to start my visits, rather behind schedule. Just as I was reversing, I saw the Mr Chalke in my mirror, hurrying towards the car and trying to catch my attention. I wound down the window and waited.

'I don't suppose you could vaccinate a couple of yearlings whilst you're here?'

Glancing at the clock and knowing they were in a field some distance away, I meant to say that I was a bit pushed for time and would add them to Thursday's list. Instead I just could not help myself. Looking him straight in the eye and smiling I replied, 'I'm sorry, Mr Chalke, but I leave the little jobs for the men.' With that I drove away.

A week later a package arrived on the equine desk. Inside was a bottle of champagne from Mr Chalke with a thank you note. From that time on we never looked back. I frequently treated his horses and then his cows. In fact we became quite friendly and I always looked forward to our chats during the course of my subsequent visits.

25

FANCY A SCOTCH?

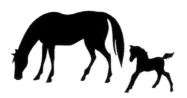

'Oh dear,' said Barbara, the practice manager. 'Mrs Houghton-Jones has a young mare that's having difficulty foaling. She wants Bob to attend but he's miles away. I don't suppose you could go?'

It was now my turn to think, 'Oh dear.' This elderly lady was a breeder of valuable Thoroughbreds and she owned a small stud on the outskirts of Salisbury. Foaling problems tend to be true emergencies. Once they go into second stage labour, mares usually give birth within twenty minutes and any departure from this often signals a real problem. Of course I would go but I knew that my arrival would be a disappointment to Mrs Houghton-Jones because Bob had looked after her horses for many years. There was the additional consideration that although I had successfully delivered hundreds of calves and several foals, I had yet to assist with a normal foaling. Those I had delivered had either been stillborn or else had serious abnormalities. I recalled the tiny foal born with his intestines hanging out that needed instant, life-saving surgery. Even sadder, I remembered helping to deliver a huge, robust foal that had only one front leg and had to be put to sleep straight away. What, I wondered, would this next visit have in store for me?

I headed off and after a few miles left the main road and followed the long, country lane leading down to the beautiful house and stud. It was my first visit and I was interested in seeing the set-up and meeting the stud manager who I knew to be very experienced and highly thought of. As I approached the stables, my heart sank as I saw the tall, young man with decidedly long arms looking out for me. If he could not deliver the foal, would I be able to? He greeted me pleasantly and went to fetch a bucket of warm water as I slipped on some clean, waterproof overalls. Then he led me to a huge foaling box and opened the long, grey metal gate at the front to let me in. And there was the young bay Thoroughbred, lying flat out in the deep straw bed, completely soaked in sweat and grunting uncomfortably.

I approached her quietly and with a few reassuring words put on a pair of arm-length, soft, plastic gloves, applied some lubricant and prepared to examine her. Just as I started, Mrs Houghton-Jones peered over the gate on tiptoe and asked me, 'Can you manage or do you need more help?'

I looked up and explained. 'I'm just about to examine the mare and will be able to answer your question if you could give me a couple of minutes please.'

Very gently I slipped my right hand inside the mare and immediately felt the foal's head. Next I should have been able to find both front feet, one slightly ahead of the other, but there was no sign of them. Reaching in a little further, I discovered the foal had its front legs folded up and as the mare strained, the foal's knees were catching on the brim of her pelvis and preventing the delivery. With my arm inside her, the mare had begun to strain forcefully so I waited until the next contraction subsided and reached forwards and cupped my hand around the tiny hoof of one of the flexed forelimbs and drew it towards me.

To my delight the leg extended easily and the hoof came to rest beside the foal's nose.

Certain that I was now going to be able to straighten the other leg and safely deliver the foal, I looked up to reassure Mrs Houghton-Jones. I was rather surprised to see only the sky over the gate instead of her anxious face as no more than a couple of minutes had passed.

'Where did she go?' I asked the stud groom.

'Oh, she couldn't wait and has gone back to the house to ring Bob.' He grinned. He explained that this was potentially an exceedingly valuable foal and when the mare had not progressed with the labour as expected, he decided to call for immediate professional assistance to be on the safe side, rather than risk wasting valuable time. It was her first foal and like many maiden mares, she had become distressed during the first stage of labour, wandering restlessly around the stable, stopping now and then to look back at her flanks and paw the ground. He had become concerned when she started to roll and sweat profusely.

I quickly explained my findings and said I was now going to straighten the second leg. As I inserted my hand for the second time and reached the flexed knee, the mare gave her next huge push and I realised that the foal was on her way into the world without any further assistance from me. She was not very big and there was plenty of room for her to emerge with the second leg still flexed. The little creature shook her head as she was delivered and I stood back and took stock to allow the mare to rest. With her bright bay coat and a small white star on her head, the foal was very pretty and would no doubt delight her anxious owner.

At about that moment, I heard a squeal of tyres and a car door slam.

'Is everything OK?' asked Bob.

'Absolutely fine,' I replied. 'I've yet to check over the mare and foal but there doesn't seem to be anything to worry about.

It wasn't my idea to call you away from whatever you were doing,' I added, 'but Mrs H-J rather jumped the gun.'

Bob grinned and as I began to tidy up, I heard Mrs H-J exclaim, 'Oh, Bob, how nice of you to come. Do come inside and have a scotch to celebrate.' With a smug glance in my direction, Bob was led off to the house and the stud groom and I burst out laughing.

I whispered, 'And a thank you and a cup of tea for the real workers would have been nice.'

My reward of course was seeing the mare and foal happily together all safe and sound. With one more backward glance at the bonny foal now struggling to her feet, I set off to catch up with my other calls.

26

A BANG ON THE HEAD

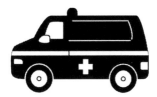

It was mid-morning and I had already been at Druid's Lodge for a couple of hours examining a selection of horses. One was lame; another had a cough and several needed their teeth rasping. Horses' teeth grow continually throughout their lifetime and need regular maintenance to prevent the development of sharp edges that can cause painful ulcers on their cheeks and tongues.

I liked working at Druid's Lodge, a livery yard with some top-quality competition horses. It was run by an amazing horsewoman with a wealth of experience and common sense. The last job on my list was to rasp the teeth of a five-year-old mare. I slipped the gag into her mouth. This is a metal device that sits on top of the front teeth and can be slowly opened, allowing you to inspect the teeth and feel safely for any sharp edges inside the mouth. The mare was a little wary but tolerant of the procedure as I inserted the rasp and carefully removed the sharp edges. I worked steadily and very soon completed the task, apart from a slight but sharp overgrowth on the front of one of the first upper molars.

The mare was a little fidgety by now so I gave her a rest and considered my options. It seemed a shame to sedate her at the client's expense when the job was 95% complete so I gently backed her into the corner of the box so she could not move away from me and continued my work. I had almost finished when she decided that enough was enough and of course the only way she could escape was to leap forwards. One moment I was looking into a horse's mouth and in the blink of an eye all I could see was a wall of chestnut hair—her belly—as she reared up on her hind legs. The next thing I felt was a front foot crashing down onto the top of my head…

I knew that I was going down and thank goodness I had followed my rule of never completely closing the stable door when treating a horse, just in case I needed to escape. As I fell I dived for the door and ended up sitting on the concrete floor outside the stable. Rather alarmingly a pool of blood began to form beside me and within a minute it was the size of a dinner plate and still spreading. I was fully conscious but very quickly the shock set in and my whole body began to tremble. I had no idea of the extent of my injury and knew the last thing I should do was to reach up with my dirty hand and explore the damage on the top of my head.

The groom who had been assigned to help me rushed off to find some assistance and came face to face with the *chef d'équipe* (team leader) of an international three-day event team who were staying at the yard for a couple of days en route to a competition. He was very capable and immediately took charge of the situation, inspecting the wound and assuring me that my skull was still intact and it was just the skin that was split open. With that reassurance and his competent kindness, rather embarrassingly my trembling gave way to uncontrolled tears. I just could not stop crying.

Shortly afterwards an ambulance with blue flashing lights arrived. I remember the paramedic asking me what day it was.

'I have no idea as it's the stud season and I work hard so one day seems to run into another,' I said. 'Can you ask me a different question?'

When we arrived at the hospital, I was put onto a trolley and taken into a private treatment room to be assessed. It was quickly established that a 10-centimetre length of skin on my head had been sliced right open, exposing the underlying bone, but that was probably the extent of the damage. Whilst waiting to be sutured, I lay quietly on the trolley and almost enjoyed a few minutes of peace in my busy life. And then I had a visitor. David, the senior partner from the farm department of the practice, popped in to see how I was. As soon as he saw the gaping hole and blood-soaked pillow, he told me not to worry about anything and to go home and rest for as long as it took me to recover.

The next visitor was a young doctor who got out his ophthalmoscope and looked into my eyes for any evidence of trauma. 'Ah,' he said with a smile. 'It's not true then. We medics always suspected that vets don't have brains but it's okay, I can see yours.'

Entering the spirit of his banter I replied, 'You must be a rubbish doctor then because if I had a brain, I wouldn't be in this situation.'

With the atmosphere lightened, we chatted away whilst he carefully cleaned and sutured my head with minimal clipping of my hair so the sutures were barely visible.

I cannot remember how I got home but I do recall the phone call from one of the equine partners later that day.

'Where's the car?' he asked.

'I left it unlocked in the yard,' I confessed.

'What! Well you'll have to go and collect it. And I hope you'll be in tomorrow.'

My head hurt by now and I was somewhat stunned by his attitude but collect the car I did.

The following day my first task was to castrate a six-year-old Thoroughbred stallion belonging to a client I had never met. It was quite a long drive away so before setting off, I tested how I felt bending over, which I would have to do underneath the sedated horse. As I doubled over, my head began to pound and I knew I should not go but as an assistant, I did as I was told in order not to upset the partners. Castrating a six-year-old stallion still standing up with sedation and local anaesthetic is not without risks to both the vet and the horse. There is no opportunity to apply a ligature to the large blood vessels and although we clamp the cord with emasculators for several minutes, the risk of haemorrhage remains. Plus, of course, there is ample opportunity for the vet to be kicked.

When I arrived I shook hands with the welcoming but business-like lady and was taken to meet my patient, a very handsome bay stallion with—yes—enormous testicles. I quickly got to work, sedating the horse and injecting local anaesthetic under the skin of the scrotum and then directly into the testicle. So far, so good. After a few minutes' wait to allow the anaesthetic to fully numb the region, I incised the scrotum, exposing the testicle. This I grasped and then applied the emasculators to the cord. With a crunch the testicle dropped to the ground and I held the emasculators in place for a few minutes before gently removing them and repeating the procedure on the other side. All went well and as I stood up, I smiled at the attentive owner.

'Well I'm pleased that's over,' I said, 'because I had a bit of an accident yesterday,' and I showed her my sutures. Instead of offering me the expected concern or sympathy, she looked very stern indeed and told me there was no way I should be at work.

'In fact,' she said, 'I'm going to phone the practice and give them a good talking-to.'

'Please don't,' I said. 'It'll only get me into trouble.'

'This is a matter of principle,' she replied. So whilst I was in the kitchen enjoying a much-needed cup of tea and biscuit, I could hear her giving someone a piece of her mind. 'How dare you...' Nothing was mentioned when I got back to the practice but I remember feeling grateful for her concern and the fact that she had my safety and welfare (as well as that of her horse) at heart.

AFRICA

O ne of the greatest privileges of being a vet is the opportunity to work with and for people from very different backgrounds. In this age of increasing concern for animal welfare, performing animals and their management are scrutinised by well-meaning people with an increasingly critical eye.

My own experiences of dealing with staff and animals in a locally based and well-known circus can only be described as an education. These people, on the whole, are professionals and in many cases their rapport with and concern for their charges is admirable. My occasional involvement has been with cases both interesting and challenging. How, I wondered, was I going to take the temperature of the tiger with diarrhoea? What could I do to stop the elephant with the sore leg from lifting me off the ground with his trunk? Should it have surprised me that the orphan baby chimp with pneumonia came into the surgery wearing a nappy and squealed in distress when I tried to take away her cuddly blanket to take an X-ray?

But nothing and no one prepared me for the zebra.

Africa was such an experienced performer that his talents

were sought from as far away as Japan. My task was to take a blood sample to establish he was free from certain infectious diseases before his journey. I envisaged a pleasant trip to the circus's winter quarters, a quick blood sample from the jugular vein as is the case with horses, a look at the other residents and a nice chat with whoever was on hand to help.

They say that zebras are amongst the most difficult to train and befriend, but Africa looked quite congenial as he was led around the corner, dwarfed by two experienced handlers. I confidently walked up to him, blood tubes in my hand, and asked if they were ready. I suppose I should have been warned by the glance that passed with raised eyebrows between the two men. As I reached out to swab Africa's neck with surgical spirit, he spun around and winded me with a single blow from his head.

Right, I thought, *let's try something else.* I looked around and spied an iron ring in a solid concrete wall so asked the two men to loop the rope from Africa's headcollar through the ring and pull his head tight against the wall. As he stood quietly now with the right side of his face against the concrete and his short body curved to the left, I reckoned it would be relatively simple to creep up to his exposed right jugular vein and draw some blood. One gentle jab and the blood would fill the attached vacutainer tube. A few seconds more and it would all be over.

That was wishful thinking. I never saw how it happened. I don't even remember blinking but two hoofs came from nowhere and delivered a resounding blow with deadly accuracy. I landed on my backside, three metres away. It didn't take many more attempts for me to realise that the zebra was far ahead of me in cunning and technique. Feeling rather embarrassed I gave up and went back to the surgery to report my failure and decide what to try next.

The following day one of my colleagues greeted me with a

smile and held up two tubes of blood labelled 'Africa'. How on earth had he achieved it?

'No problem at all,' he told me. The zebra had apparently put up no resistance.

Intrigued, I enquired, 'Just how did you manage that?'

'Some of us have it and some of us don't,' he said as he disappeared out through the door.

'Hmmm.' I could not believe that it was that simple. Later on in the day, however, one of the farm vets said he had heard I had experienced a bit of trouble with a zebra. I laughed and admitted it but confessed to having no idea how the other vet managed successfully.

'Didn't he tell you he borrowed the dart gun?'

Aha, so that was it! More experienced in the art of *not* handling zebras, he had arrived at the circus with a dart gun and a suitable dose of anaesthetic. One moment Africa was relaxing in his stable and a few minutes later he was snoring away in the straw. Taking the blood was painless for everyone apart from me who was black and blue from the previous day's antics.

Once the mission was accomplished, the antidote was given and within minutes the surprised animal was back on his feet, wondering what had happened.

That is the other great thing about our job: you never stop learning—sometimes the hard way.

28

A NEW DIRECTION AND THE PATTER
OF TINY FEET

Three years after I arrived in Salisbury, I realised I was beginning to burn out. When I had a health scare (a large but thankfully benign breast tumour), it made me take a step back and look at my life. The equine vets in the practice were relatively young and there was no prospect of a partnership, so I took the rather scary decision to resign. I had plenty of projects in mind and thanks to my friend Liz, had a publisher lined up for a book that was far from completion. Liz had noticed that there were no veterinary books for the horse owner that explained the various equine ailments in some detail but used everyday language that was easily understood. She had continually pestered me to start writing and eventually I managed a few chapters, starting at 11 p.m. and working into the early hours. Liz submitted them to the publisher, J.A.Allen, who immediately offered us a contract for the first edition of *The Veterinary Care of the Horse*.

I remember my first day of not working as a vet. It was strange but nice to see my house in daylight but initially the hours seemed to stretch endlessly ahead like a great empty space. I had a lovely horse to ride by now, but I was used to doing that at 6 a.m. and being on the road by 8 a.m. I set up my typewriter (I did not have a computer then) on the dining room table, made a list of the book's contents and started to write. Once I got my head around this new way of life, I likened it to being in a ploughed field. I felt as though I lived in the furrow where I beavered away, concentrating intently on my work, and every now and then I popped up to rejoin the real world and be sociable, only to dive back down into the furrow to begin the next chapter or topic.

It was good to cross subjects off the list and then post them to Liz who would edit them and tell me off if I used language that was too technical. All very different from the veterinary life that I loved, so when one of the senior farm vets phoned from the practice I had recently left and asked me to join their team for five months, I welcomed the escape and willingly donned the wellington boots and green overalls. I helped out with the farm work whilst the student who was to be their next assistant sat his finals.

When he qualified and took up his position, I found myself back at the dining room table. By now the book was coming on nicely and I was enjoying my new hobby of photography to illustrate it. Then two things happened. Firstly, I received a telephone call from the small animal department of the same practice, asking if I could step in as a locum as their young assistant had left suddenly. This was of interest to me as I could continue writing and still be part of a good veterinary team, with hours to suit us both. Secondly, shortly after I accepted, I discovered I was expecting my first child. We agreed that I would join the team as planned but not do any routine surgery to minimise my exposure to anaesthetic gases. Working with Gerry, Lynne, Margaret and Sam for the next few months was a great experience.

On my very first day, I happily donned a starched, white coat and hung a stethoscope around my neck, ready for the challenge. Having not treated any small animals for three years, I was particularly concerned that I might miss an important sign that could delay a diagnosis at the patient's expense. The day started well: a puppy to check over and vaccinate, a cat with an abscess and a dog with sore ears. But then a large and subdued-looking German shepherd dog came through the door with his concerned owner. Bonzo had been fine yesterday, eating normally and enjoying his walks, but late in the evening he started vomiting. This had continued all night and although it was only 9:30 a.m., he had already been sick several times that morning.

I went through the usual questions: Had he eaten any rubbish? Did he chew stones? Could he have swallowed a toy? All negative and examining him did not throw any light on the situation either. This left me with two choices: advise the owner to starve him for 24 hours with small drinks of water—and I would inject him with a drug to stop the vomiting—or admit him for an X-ray in case there was an obstruction or foreign body. Help! My first day and some clinical instinct warned me that this dog needed further investigation. I suspected that my new team might think I was being over-cautious if I sent him across to the operations area. What to do? There was no real choice as I would have felt uncomfortable about sending him home so I admitted Bonzo and handed him over to one of the nurses.

It was a nice tradition in this practice that we stopped at 10:30 a.m. for coffee with the whole small animal team if at all possible. This gave us time to discuss any cases and just to chat. Thus it was no surprise when Gerry took me to one side and kindly explained that in most cases they would normally leave it for 24 hours before admitting a vomiting dog for an X-ray. Feeling a bit of an idiot and somewhat embarrassed, I went back to the consulting rooms to continue the morning appointments. Then at lunchtime, one of the nurses came and told me that

Gerry wanted me to go back over to the operating theatre. Uh-oh, had I done something else wrong?

Gerry's face was serious as he switched on the X-ray viewing box and put up a radiograph of a dog's abdomen. 'Now, what do you think is going on here?' he asked. As I studied the image, a strikingly large, black circle stood out in the region of the dog's stomach, looking suspiciously like a ball. With the beginnings of a smile, I looked up at Gerry and asked, 'Is that my earlier patient?'

'It certainly is. Well done and welcome to the team.'

Later that day the ball was successfully removed and Bonzo quickly made a full recovery. He had provided me with a big confidence boost on my very first day and helped me feel that I deserved my place in the team.

* * *

Towards the end of my time as a small animal vet, we went through a run of caesareans needing to be done late on a Monday night and three in a row had been chocolate Labradors. And sure enough it was 11 p.m. when the phone call came asking me to go to the surgery as a Labrador was having difficulty whelping. Missy was a lovely dog, obviously full of pups and suffering from primary uterine inertia, which is when the uterus fails to contract effectively to push the pups out. She had been restless and panting all evening, with a few weak contractions, but the labour had not progressed. With sterile gloves and a lubricated finger, I quickly established that there was no obstruction and administered an injection of oxytocin to stimulate the uterus to contract. We popped her into a quiet kennel with a comfy bed and waited to see if the treatment would work, whilst at the same time preparing to operate, just in case.

When it became apparent that Missy needed a caesarean, the

nurse and I gently lifted her onto the table. With the nurse talking to her the whole time, I inserted an intravenous catheter and gave her the anaesthetic. Speed and efficiency are important from this stage onwards to ensure the puppies receive as little of the anaesthetic as possible. The nurse clipped and scrubbed up Missy's abdomen whilst I donned a surgical gown and scrubbed up. The operation proceeded well and one by one, eleven small, chocolate puppies were delivered without complication. By the end of the procedure, reaching over my own baby bump had taken its toll on my aching back and I considered the possibility that now was perhaps the time to give up emergency surgery.

I started to suture the uterus and observed a small bleed that started when I removed the last puppy and placenta. I was not at this stage concerned, thinking that it would quickly be brought under control. But that was not to be. I did everything I could both medically and surgically to get the bleeding under control, but my next phone call was to the owner, advising her that I needed to spay Missy to stop the haemorrhage and seeking permission to go ahead. The owner was a lovely lady, who really cared for her dog, and she told me to do whatever was necessary.

Thus at 1 a.m., I started to spay Missy. I ligated and detached the first ovary and that was when she stopped breathing. The nurse and I went into resuscitation mode straight away, each of us knowing our roles. I ventilated Missy manually with oxygen whilst the nurse fetched the emergency drugs for me to insert into the intravenous line that was already in place. We watched and we waited and still nothing. In my head I was already having a ghastly conversation explaining to the owner that her dog had died on the operating table. A couple of minutes passed and my heart truly began to sink, when suddenly, Missy took a tiny breath and her pulse, which had been horribly faint, became stronger. Within a few more minutes, she was breathing normally and I was able to recommence the surgery. This was straightforward, without further complication, and as soon as she came round we were able to phone her owner so she could collect Missy and her puppies.

I would like to say that that was the end of the story but more drama was yet to come. At 3:30 a.m. I collapsed into bed but within just a few minutes, a fleeting concern crossed my mind. When we stopped to resuscitate Missy, I had attached a pair of Allis tissue forceps to the stump of the ovary I had just removed—a common practice so it could be relocated easily to check for any bleeding before she was sewn up. With large dogs it is quite possible for the forceps to almost disappear from sight and in that moment of horror, I could not remember if in the heat of the situation I had gone back in to remove them. Oh my goodness, I was now in a complete panic. They were very unlikely to cause any harm in the short term but how on earth was I going to tell the owner whose dog had nearly died under the anaesthetic that her pet needed another one to remove the forceps that I had left inside her? No sleep for me that night and I realised that when Missy came in for her post-operative check in the morning, I would have to X-ray her abdomen to see if the forceps were there.

By 8 a.m. I was back in the operating theatre, making plans for the day and confiding my concern to the nurse who had worked with me throughout the night. At this point she stopped what she was doing and a huge smile spread across her face. 'There's no need to worry, Sue. Counting the instruments is my job and I can assure you that we have the same number that we started with.' What a relief and not for the first time did I thank my lucky stars for having such wonderful and professional nurses to keep us vets in order.

* * *

Not long after that night, on the morning of September 13th 1991, I went into labour. Two days later the baby had still not arrived and eventually at 3:44 a.m. on 16th September, my son, Alex, was born by emergency caesarean.

Alex was a wonderfully contented baby and after a while I went back to work part-time. In 1992 our book was published and Liz and I were very proud when it became J.A.Allen's top seller of the year. The nice thing about working for a small publisher is that they know their authors personally and make them feel special. We were regularly invited to attend their Christmas parties where we met other authors and had an insight into a world that was very different from our own. When the sales reached 25,000 and then 30,000 and 40,000 copies, we were presented with specially engraved glass goblets to mark the occasion.

For the next three and a half years, I juggled family life with small animal veterinary work and then on February 8th 1995 my daughter, Laura, was born. I was delighted to have a little girl and felt that our family was now complete. When I returned home and the health visitor called, she said our house had a very happy and special atmosphere.

Sadly this did not last for long and just a few weeks later, my world fell apart when I unexpectedly became a single parent.

29

ANOTHER BEGINNING

L ife was very different following John's sudden departure but I did the best I could with the support of my friends and family. Luckily Alex and Laura were happy and adaptable children and seemed unperturbed as I changed jobs a couple of times and tried to establish a better balance between work and home life. In the end though, work always seemed to have first call on my time and to start with it was also my escape from the difficulty and sadness of being a single parent. Even setting up an equine practice with a colleague and job sharing did not solve the problem as the cost of the necessary childcare and babysitters was prohibitive and left me feeling the balance was still wrong.

The solution came as the result of an unfortunate accident and was definitely a silver lining to what had seemed a large, black cloud at the time. When Alex was a baby, I fell off a horse at high speed and landed headfirst at the bottom of a fence. The vertebrae in my neck were compressed and I was severely concussed. I had a couple of physiotherapy sessions and recovered well but six weeks later I began to experience ferocious pins and needles in my right arm when it was in certain positions. This progressed to not being able to turn my neck at all to the right and then it only took another small jolt for my back to seize up as well.

The arthritic changes in my neck caused pressure on the cervical nerve roots and I developed a condition called complex regional pain syndrome which gave me cold, slightly swollen and very painful hands. I consulted my GP who referred me to an orthopaedic surgeon, a neurologist and rheumatologists, all of whom did their best but were unable to do much to help. The symptoms were variable from day to day and did not respond to any of the painkillers that I was prescribed. I managed to cope with the small animal work thanks to the assistance of our excellent nurses but knew that a return to equine work was out of the question. I tried physiotherapy, chiropractic and the Alexander technique, but nothing made much difference.

Then my luck changed. I was having a particularly bad day and telephoned my GP to ask if there was something else I could try. I could not accept that I was going to feel this uncomfortable for the rest of my life. He had just returned from a weekend course on acupuncture and thought it might help me. He referred me to an experienced practitioner and that was the beginning of my recovery. Will explained that my muscles had become very tight and irritable. He only had to feel my neck and back and the muscles spontaneously jumped beneath his fingers. I had developed myofascial pain syndrome. With weekly acupuncture treatments, my muscles gradually relaxed and lengthened, allowing greater range of movement and much-reduced pain. I will never forget the moment after the fifth treatment when I realised that for about an hour nothing hurt. By the eleventh treatment, I was pain-free for most of the day. I then had the confidence to have further chiropractic treatment and thanks to the skills of the amazing chiropractic team of Nigel, Jenny and Alex, gained more movement of my neck.

I had been released from a long period of pain and

immobility and felt as though I had been given my life back. I wanted to tell everyone about this wonderful treatment. It did not take long before I began to think about all of the horses and ponies with back and neck pain that did not recover with rest and painkillers. Surely they too could benefit from acupuncture? The rest, as the saying goes, is history. I trained over a period of a year with the International Veterinary Acupuncture Society and in January 2000 passed my exams and became a certified veterinary acupuncturist. Then on April 1st 2002, I started my own Equine Acupuncture Referral Practice. Finally, I had found the way to balance the needs of my growing children whilst still doing a fulfilling and worthwhile job that I loved.

30

MY NEW PRACTICE

On April 2nd, I set off on my visits with a spring in my step. The sun shone as I drove across the New Forest feeling good about my new way of life. I had been lucky enough to find Kayte, a wonderful lady, to work part time and help me with the children, my business, the animals and even cook us all delicious meals.

The following day, as I walked into the spring meeting of the Association of British Veterinary Acupuncturists at the ICC in Birmingham, I was greeted by a group of colleagues who asked if I would stand for election as secretary. Although I am not a committee person, the timing seemed right so I accepted. When I stood up to address the meeting and mentioned I had just established an equine acupuncture practice, there was a collective gasp of disbelief that I would have enough work to make it a successful business. However, this was the beginning of a new era and others have now followed my lead.

Even though acupuncture had worked so well for my injuries, I was continually delighted at just how effective it was when I first started treating horses. Week after week I would be greeted by smiling owners and comments such as 'I'd forgotten what a sweet-natured horse he used to be' as the horses experienced the muscle relaxation and pain relief that restored their good humour. Another benefit was the improvement in their performance and as other horse owners observed this, they asked for their horses to be examined. I was fortunate in never having to advertise as the results spoke for themselves and in the summer months, I would often have a waiting list.

Ninety-nine per cent of my patients were horses and ponies but I would also treat donkeys and cows if requested. I enjoyed the variety of work immensely. To begin with I saw a lot of horses as the last resort, when every other treatment had failed. I was happy to take on these cases and by far the majority were saved and went on to lead useful lives. Then gradually I began to see horses earlier and treat elite performance horses to keep them at the peak of fitness. Detecting and treating minor injuries at an early stage could prevent them from developing into more serious problems that were likely to cause lameness and necessitate their withdrawal from competitions or finish their careers. I took great pleasure from watching them race, event and perform dressage successfully and in some cases go on to represent their country in international events. It was a privilege to attend some of these events and be on hand to provide help if necessary.

Inevitably there are always cases that are particularly memorable for one reason or another and here are just a few.

31

THE POWER OF TRADITIONAL CHINESE MEDICINE (TCM)

A small, fifteen-year-old chestnut mare that was one of my very first acupuncture patients will always stand out in my memory. Cindy had been off her food and looking dejected for a few days when her owner called the vet. A colleague had examined her thoroughly but could find nothing to explain her malaise so took some blood tests. These too were normal with the exception of a slightly depressed white cell count, suggesting she may be recovering from a virus. The vet treated her with multivitamins to give her a boost but still she refused her hard food and hay. She lived out in a field with a wooden shelter that had a deep bed of clean, dry straw. Cindy was always susceptible to feeling the cold and although she was protected from the wind and rain with a warm, comfortable rug, she had spent most of the day inside the shelter for the last week. She only came out briefly to nibble the poor winter grass and at this stage I was asked if I could do anything to help her.

Keen to try the TCM that I had spent so much time trying to understand and learn, I arranged an appointment and repeated the clinical examination. I checked her mouth and teeth, looked at her mucous membranes, listened to her heart and gut sounds with a stethoscope and then did an internal examination, all with no untoward findings. Her temperature was lower than normal and from samples of dung and blood examined the previous week, we knew she did not have a problem with internal parasites. This was a little mare that I had known for several years and there was no doubt that her coat looked dry and lacklustre and she had an air of general lethargy. I asked her owner to fetch me a bucket containing some tasty pasture mix and offered it to Cindy. Just as reported, she turned her face away and was not interested in even trying it.

I have subsequently found that where Western medicine does not have the answers, TCM usually provides a treatment option. After taking a detailed history, I gently felt Cindy all over from head to tail to identify whether she had any tender spots. I was intrigued but not surprised when the four sensitive points on her body correlated with those I would expect to find on a patient that was not eating and had recently been exposed to cold, wet and windy conditions. We moved her into a stable and by now quite a crowd had gathered to see what this unfamiliar treatment involved. Cindy stood quietly as I gently inserted the needles into points known to stimulate appetite and gut activity. I used 21 needles and as the treatment progressed, she gradually lowered her head and became more and more sleepy. I warmed some of the stainless steel needles with a stick of burning moxa (which looks like a burning cigar) as she dozed quietly, seemingly oblivious to the hushed crowd of people watching.

Whilst the treatment proceeded, I explained to those interested that in TCM, Cindy was experiencing a generalised Qi (pronounced 'chee') deficiency that had allowed the invasion of Pathogenic Cold. The Qi deficiency was probably the result of many factors, including her advancing years, the fact that she had produced and raised a strong healthy foal the previous year and the poor quality of the grass and hay available to her. This gave rise to her reduced appetite, sensitivity to the cold and depressed immune system, making her susceptible to a viral infection, which in TCM is a Cold pathogen.

The points that I selected would also boost her immune system and the moxa warmed the points up to expel the Cold. Although it might sound far-fetched using points on her body to influence her health, the neurophysiology is well understood. Nerve fibres from internal organs pass into the spinal cord very close to those from localised areas of skin on either the back or the abdominal wall. They are very closely associated with each other and share the same pathways to the brain, with the result that disease in an internal organ can refer pain to specific sites on the body. A well-known example of this in humans is the pain often experienced in the left arm when someone is having a heart attack and McBurney's point, low on the right side of the abdomen, that is tender to touch when the patient has appendicitis. The same nerve pathways also account for the fact that stimulating a particular point on the body surface can influence the function of an internal organ.

After fifteen to twenty minutes of deep relaxation, Cindy lifted her head and became alert. I removed the needles and we led her outside. Within a short space of time, she passed some droppings and her increased gut sounds were clearly audible to all of us so I asked her owner to go and make up a small feed. The mare recognised the familiar sounds coming from the feed shed and stared intently at the door, pawing the ground with her ears pricked. As the food was brought out, she showed a healthy excitement and immediately began to eat, not stopping until it was all gone.

Moments such as this make me deeply respectful of and excited by the power of acupuncture. Cindy had refused concentrates for the previous three weeks and turned away from the bucket only half an hour before. For the next few days, she continued to eat her feeds but still would not eat the hay. Following a second treatment a week later, her appetite and demeanour returned to normal.

* * *

When I still worked in general equine practice, I also found acupuncture particularly helpful as part of the treatment for selected cases where the horse was experiencing colicky pain. I generally assigned these patients into one of three groups. There were the straightforward, spasmodic colics and horses with impactions of their large bowel that usually responded well to the appropriate medical therapy. Then there were those that required immediate surgery or euthanasia. The third group, however, required careful monitoring. They often had reduced gut activity and powerful intravenous painkillers did not completely abolish their pain. At the time of examination, they did not require surgery but the situation could change quickly and the sooner any deterioration was recognised, the greater the horse's chance of survival. In these cases, I would often stay a while and monitor the horse, particularly if the call was some distance from the surgery. In other instances, a second visit was needed later in the day.

It was one evening when I was chatting to the owner of a horse that continued to experience discomfort that I asked for the first time if I could try some acupuncture. The two-year-old gelding showed no objection as I inserted eleven needles and almost immediately we could hear rumbling sounds from his abdomen. He stopped pawing the ground and started to nibble some hay and within five minutes was back to his normal self. Since then I have used acupuncture together with conventional treatment to speed the recovery of dozens of horses and ponies and spare them the misery of continuing tummy ache and their owners from hours of worry. How lucky and privileged I feel to have discovered this powerful addition to the treatments I can offer.

32

THE RUNAWAY COW

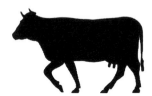

I have always had a special liking for cows as they are gentle and inquisitive creatures. In the early days of mixed practice, when I was on duty and the phone rang, I would wait in suspense for the night telephone lady to tell me which species of animal was in trouble. If the visit was to see a cow, there was a wide spectrum of possible problems including injuries, acute mastitis, metabolic upsets and calving difficulties. Nowadays the only cows I tend to see are those who cannot get up after calving due to severe bruising or nerve damage from giving birth, or cows that have serious injuries from slipping on concrete yards.

And so it was that our local dairy farmer asked me to come and give some acupuncture to a cow that was still unable to stand, having calved four days earlier. It was always a pleasure to help David as on most days for the last twenty years he had waved to me as I passed his farm on the way to work. If I was a little early and turned up as the cows were crossing the road from the field to the dairy, he would joke that I was the only person he ever stopped the cows to let through. I mistakenly thought it was because he realised the value of my work and that I may be in a hurry, but years later he explained that with toast in one of my hands and coffee in the other, he considered it to be the safest course of action. We also had a good arrangement about payment. He was not given a vet's bill and I did not pay to have the grass in my field cut or my muck heap removed.

It was a busy day and I could not give an exact time of arrival so the dairyman was nowhere to be seen when I arrived. The cow, however, was sitting on a deep and comfortable straw bed with her calf nearby. She was chewing her cud and seemed quite unperturbed as I checked her over. Her temperature, pulse, colour, udder and limbs were all fine and as I had spoken to the farm vet who had examined her the previous day, I knew that her blood samples were normal too. She had been prescribed anti-inflammatory and pain-relieving medicines but was still unable to stand. On a number of occasions, she made a huge effort and almost made it but then her legs crumpled beneath her.

I brushed the bits of straw off her back and inserted the acupuncture needles at sites selected to give maximum pain relief to cows with pelvic injuries. I then attached the electrodes from a battery-operated electroacupuncture unit to four of the needles. Once the machine was turned on, I increased the intensity of stimulation so the needles could just be seen to move at two alternating frequencies. This is not uncomfortable for the patient; it just gives a vibrating sensation but it is a more powerful treatment than using the needles alone. The cow sat quietly throughout, her dark brown eyes following the antics of her playful calf, and as we sat there together, the dairyman arrived. We chatted about her management over the next few days and I arranged to call in the next day and repeat the treatment if she was still not up.

The following day there was a note on the gate of the pen saying the cow had briefly stood up during the previous evening but was not in a hurry to try again. After I'd checked her over once more, I repeated the treatment and patted her, saying that if she wanted to avoid a third time then she had better be up and out of there by the time I next called. Late the same afternoon, I stopped at the farm on my way home and was delighted to see the door of the pen wide open and the cow grazing with her calf in the nearby field. Job done and I thought that was the end of the story.

Two months later it was the afternoon of the annual Farley fete. The sun was shining and the activities were in full swing. Skittle competitions, coconuts to knock out of their hoops and raffle stalls attracted custom under the bunting that fluttered in the breeze. The brass band was playing and the fun dog show—for which I was the judge—was commencing shortly. I saw David's daughter gesticulating at me from her post at the cake stall and made my way over to say hello. She had always taken a big interest in the dairy farm and I could only just hear her say something about the cow I treated, as the band was so close by.

'Oh yes,' I said. 'She's OK, isn't she?'

'Yes, but did you hear what happened when she rejoined the rest of the herd?' She paused. 'For two days she trotted non-stop around the edge of the field and went through the fence twice, letting the other cows out in the process. Dad reckoned you left your electroacupuncture unit on the racehorse setting and not the cow one.'

The truth of course is that being separated from her calf probably unsettled the cow but to this day it is a village joke that my acupuncture not only got the cow up but made her think she was a racehorse.

33

THE IMPORTANCE OF TEAM WORK

During the course of my work, I made some special friends and met a number of other professionals for whom I developed enormous respect. And so it was with Amanda, a veterinary physiotherapist, who had travelled extensively with the British three-day event team. I remember feeling very uncomfortable in my early days whenever I asked her to come and treat a horse with me. She was so knowledgeable and infinitely better than I was at finding the sore spots on the animal. In fact I began to dread these meetings, always on the back foot, feeling challenged and ignorant. There was only one way to tackle this and that was to ask for her help so I could examine my patients and find the source of their pain with the same ease. As well as being an excellent therapist, she was a good teacher and it was not long before I palpated my patients with confidence.

After that we began to work together, combining our individual skills, and I was very pleased when she asked me to be the attending vet for monthly osteopathy clinics. This was a window of opportunity for me to observe the skills of a highly respected osteopath. People brought their horses from far and wide for his attention, with several well-known riders amongst them.

And then Amanda introduced me to our country's leading three-day-event rider and suggested that I should treat a number of his horses. She had worked as his equine physiotherapist for many years, travelling with him to major events, and she thought that the horses would benefit from acupuncture.

Well, this was my dream. Three-day eventing had been my passion since I was a child and the opportunity to treat some of the world's top horses was very special. I was excited and anxious in equal measure but it was a challenge I embraced with enthusiasm. On my first visit to the yard, I loved walking along the rows of stables in the light, airy barns, admiring the array of elite horses. To me, three-day eventing is the ultimate equestrian sport. On day one they have to perform a dressage test in an arena with letters at various points around the perimeter. The test includes movements at walk, trot and canter, requiring accuracy and complete obedience, as well as style and athleticism. The arena is surrounded with spectator stands and on occasions the atmosphere can be too electric for a supremely fit and lively horse to perform their best.

Day two is a cross-country course over four miles in length with at least 40 obstacles to be jumped, testing the fitness and courage of the horse and the trust and mutual understanding between horse and rider. To have any chance of being placed in the competition, they need to jump clear and preferably within the tight time allowed. On the third day, which is traditionally a Sunday, the horses that have come safely through the cross country have to pass a vet's inspection to see if they are sound and fit enough to complete the third phase—the show jumping —a final test of accuracy and ability following the demands of the day before.

The Sunday morning vet's inspection is a big event, open to

the public, who fill the stands to overflowing. The competitors present their horses to the vet and the Ground Jury and additional interest is provided as there is a prize for the best-dressed rider. With horse and rider under scrutiny, the atmosphere is hushed and expectant as each horse is trotted up with a burst of applause if the horse is accepted.

For several years, Amanda and I were part of the team whose task it was to make sure the horses in our care were fit and sound enough to pass the vet's inspection and hopefully go on to jump clear in the show jumping. We would watch the cross country with fingers crossed and our hearts racing, hoping for a fast, clear round but most of all for the horses' safe return. Both of us were involved in the preparation of the horses in the months building up to the event, but the intensive work began the moment the rider dismounted after the cross country. Each horse was cooled down with gallons of water and walked around to prevent stiffness setting in. One of the many vets on duty at the event then inspected the horse and watched it trot up as another check on their welfare.

Back at the stables, there was tight security as everyone quietly went about the business of caring for their horses. Grooms, physiotherapists, chiropractors, farriers and vets worked as a team with each horse and there was great camaraderie between the different teams. It always gave me a thrill and real sense of privilege to be so close to so many of the world's top horses and riders and I was amazed at how calm and relaxed the horses were away from home and their usual routine.

Once the horses were rested and when we felt the time was right, the groom and I quietly got on and treated them with acupuncture, having obtained permission from the appropriate authority. This helped to ease tired and tight muscles and alleviate any stiffness before they were left in peace to rest for the night.

The next morning we would be up bright and early preparing for the vet's inspection. Thankfully over the years our horses always passed, and I was very proud to have been a small part of the winning team at Badminton and Burghley horse trials on several occasions.

NUTTY

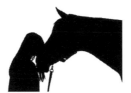

E very now and then I come across a special horse that touches my heart. Nutty was a dark bay Thoroughbred who had raced as a youngster. As a result of his endeavours, he had developed arthritic changes in his fetlocks and hocks that brought an end to his racing career. Luckily for him he was retired and then at the age of sixteen was given to Felicity who had always had a soft spot for him. Whatever Nutty needed, he was given and Felicity worked hard to provide for him. As the years passed, Nutty began to develop painful spasms in the muscles on the left side of his back, probably from years of holding himself abnormally to compensate for his stiff limbs. As he showed little response to the prescribed pain-relieving drugs, Felicity wanted to see if acupuncture would help him so she contacted me.

Nutty was a sweet-natured and kind horse but he became agitated if confined in a small space. I usually ask for my acupuncture patients to be stabled the night before the first examination to ensure that they are clean and dry. Nutty, however, was waiting for me in a large field with several companions. He was a gentle giant and trotted over when we called him. All of his lower limb joints were thickened and he appeared to be lame on three of his four legs. Once his headcollar was on, I was able to establish that his neck muscles were a little tight and sore but when I gently felt along the left side of his back he grunted and dipped down to avoid my touch; the muscles of his hindquarters were similarly painful.

With such severe muscle spasm, I opted to give Nutty a little sedation so he remained relaxed for his first treatment, especially as his equine companions had gathered around to see what was going on. The last thing I wanted was for him to suddenly decide he had had enough and to gallop off, leaving a trail of needles in his wake. I had to smile at finding myself performing acupuncture on a sensitive Thoroughbred in the middle of a twenty-acre field whilst his friends nudged at my pockets and turned out the holdall containing my equipment. Every now and then, they squabbled amongst themselves and shot off with a display of heels and swish of their tails. Nutty stood calmly and visibly relaxed as the treatment proceeded. The long muscles of his back twitched repeatedly in response to the needling, always an encouraging sign. Optimistic that he would respond as hoped, I made an appointment to see him in several days' time.

Most horses feel considerably better after the first treatment but may not show an improvement in performance until they have been treated for a second time. Our aim with Nutty was simply to make him as comfortable as possible all over. A week later he was definitely more mobile and happier in himself but there was little, if any, improvement in his back muscles, so this time I treated him with electroacupuncture. He became profoundly relaxed and we realised that it was no longer necessary give any sedation as he seemed to sense that we were helping him. After the fourth treatment, we were delighted that he was no longer lame when trotted up, but I was a little disappointed that his back was still sore.

It is a testament to Felicity's determination and faith that she was willing to continue and the next time I saw Nutty there was a big improvement. It took eight treatments for the pain to go altogether and from then on I saw him once a month for a while and then we were able to extend the gap between treatments to three months.

I have very fond memories of treating this patient and gentle horse. On one occasion when it was pouring with rain, I urged Felicity to let me try to examine him in the stable. Just as she predicted, he was claustrophobic and would not settle, so we ended up outside with Felicity lifting his waterproof rug so I could move underneath and insert the needles. From then on our visits were planned around the weather forecast.

I particularly remember one summer's day when I arrived early and found Nutty and his friends were now sharing an even larger field with some young cattle. Felicity rented the fields from a farmer so the horses had to move around to fit in with his plans. We left my bag of equipment outside the field gate and set off to catch Nutty and bring him over for his treatment. It was quite a long walk and as we returned, I could see that the cattle were playing with something. To my horror it was my bag, and all of my sterile equipment and the bottles of expensive sedative were being tossed around and rolled in the cow pats which they had produced in their excitement. It turned out that part of the metal gate was broken and they had managed to reach through and grasp the bag. At these moments there is no point in getting cross as the damage was done. It was just another expensive lesson learnt.

Nutty is sadly no longer with us but there is no doubt that he was pain-free and enjoyed the best of care in his twilight years thanks to his owner. He will always be remembered as a special horse.

PART TWO

35

THE DAY EVERYTHING CHANGED

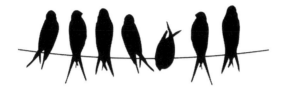

The morning of October 15th 2009 began well and I arrived bright and early at 8 a.m. to see one of my favourite horses. By far the majority of my patients receive treatment so they can run faster, jump higher or perform dressage more fluently for their owners. But not Finn. At 19 years old, this lovely grey Thoroughbred had aged beyond his years with arthritis that had prevented him from being ridden for some time. Much loved by his owner who spent her savings on keeping him comfortable and happy, he pottered around the field by day with his friends and came into his stable at night. With an acupuncture treatment every couple of months, he was kept as mobile as possible, able to enjoy playing with his companions and a daily roll in the pasture.

Finn loved his acupuncture. As his owner had her leg in plaster following an operation and was unable to hold him, he enjoyed munching some hay tied up to the fence whilst I treated him. Spending an hour examining and treating this companionable horse never failed to make me feel privileged and was always a good start to the day.

The rest of the morning passed with a couple more visits.

Nothing too serious or taxing and by 3 p.m. I headed back to Salisbury for a routine follow-up appointment at Salisbury District Hospital. Earlier in the year I had had a bit of a scare with a fast-growing thyroid cyst. It was successfully drained and I had recently had an ultrasound examination, which showed no sign of recurrence. As I drove through Bishopdown, I felt quite relaxed, confident that today I would be signed off.

I then remembered that Miss Aertssen, my consultant, was also the breast surgeon so perhaps now would be a good time to give myself a quick check, something I always have to steel myself for, having found that benign tumour around twenty years earlier. I did not expect to find anything untoward so when a large, hard lump seemed to jump into my hand, a black stab of fear instantly coursed through my body and my whole world turned upside down. I felt sick and terrified as I checked again. There was no doubt. And I knew for certain that this time, it was cancer. Sheer panic washed over me as my thoughts ran away. If it was that big in such a short time, where else had it spread? Then the question that every mother in this situation asks: 'What about my children?'

Still terrified, I made my way to the reception of surgical outpatients, wondering what to do. Would Miss Aertssen be prepared to examine me that day or would I have an agonising wait for a future appointment? I explained my predicament to the busy receptionist and the kindly lady told me to take a seat whilst she went and had a word with Miss Aertssen. I waited with waves of fear still surging through my body until I felt the receptionist place her hand gently and reassuringly on my shoulder, with the message that it was all in hand and I would be seen that day. Thank goodness. What a relief to pass the responsibility for managing this nightmare over to someone else.

It was not long before I was called through and examined by a young registrar who tried to be reassuring. Then Miss

Aertssen appeared and in her kind and efficient way examined me and explained that further investigations were necessary to determine the nature of the lump. She sent me for a mammogram and from there to the ultrasound department. As I lay on the bed, I could see the scattered calcium deposits on the screen that indicated it was indeed a tumour. The young doctor and the nurse answered my questions honestly and said they would take some biopsies right away.

The doctor injected me with some local anaesthetic so I felt no discomfort as he used the ultrasound to guide the biopsy needle to the suspicious-looking area. The procedure was soon completed with only slight tugging sensations as the samples of tissue were expertly removed. I was warned to expect some mild discomfort and bruising for a few days and sent back to the waiting room.

By now it was 5 p.m. and the hustle and bustle of the busy department had subsided. As I sat alone, a sense of gratitude and relief replaced my panic. In less than two hours, I had found the lump, had a mammogram and several biopsies and was now well and truly in the system. I was also being well looked after. A nurse came and took me back to see Miss Aertssen who gently went through the various possibilities but warned me to expect bad news. Armed with a handful of booklets, I was escorted back to reception to make an appointment to receive the biopsy results in a week. Until this moment I had been in a state of stunned shock but now the potential enormity of my situation hit me and silent tears began to slip down my cheeks.

Shirley, one of the two very special, breast-care nurses, took me into a side room and made me a cup of tea. I shared my concerns about being a single parent with two dependent children. Alex had just started his A-level year at school and Laura was only fourteen. I wasn't quite sure how I was going to manage. Then what of my business? My clients and patients? Who would care for them if I was unable to work? I had worked so hard to establish my practice and at that moment I felt overwhelmed.

It was dark by the time I left the hospital and walked to the car park. There was now the question of who to share this news with. I felt burdened with a dark secret and did not want to inflict it on any of my friends or family, all of whom had enough worries of their own. Nor did I want to tell Alex and Laura. Half term was approaching and they were going away with their father. I wanted to tell them when I would be around to answer any questions and reassure them. In any case I did not have the whole picture yet. Maybe, just maybe, there would be nothing to worry them.

In the end I shared the news with my two sisters, Jane and Judy, both of whom were wonderfully supportive, just as I knew they would be. Judy is a nurse with considerable experience of cancer patients and Jane is a pharmacist who had experienced breast cancer herself. What a backup team! Fortified with their compassion and support, I felt ready to embrace the next step.

36

THE DAYS THAT FOLLOWED

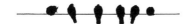

That was Thursday and by Saturday I felt in limbo, awaiting the biopsy results. I had been here before but this time it was different. 'Be prepared for bad news,' Miss Aertssen had said. The question was 'How bad?' In five days I would find out.

I had coffee in Salisbury with my best friend Izzy. I had not told her yet because I knew she would be upset. Anyone who has cancer knows how difficult it is to spoil other people's days and watch their faces as you tell them your news.

As I stepped out of Reeve the baker into the market square, I felt cocooned in a rather detached and private place with my secret. I saw the world differently. I felt completely well, not the slightest bit ill. I stood still for a moment, watching as people passed me by, going about the business of their daily lives, and I smiled at them. Most smiled back. I wondered if any of them had cancer but did not know it yet. And then felt guilty for the thought.

Whilst in Tesco my mobile phone rang with an enquiry from a potential new client. I did not know what to say. Should I be taking on new patients? I decided to be positive and book them in and then treated myself to some flowers. During this week of uncertainty, I carried on working as normal. My job requires total focus so this was definitely a good way to pass the time. When I was with the horses, the cloud hovering over me receded from my conscious thoughts. I did confide in one or two of my regular clients as I knew that major surgery was imminent, and their unequivocal support and concern was a great help. I received many hugs.

I spent the evening with another good friend, Rosie. As she was in plaster with a broken ankle, I took an Indian takeaway to her house and we had a lovely time watching TV and chatting whilst sharing a bottle of sparkling wine. Her gentle yellow Labrador, Alice, sat with us and hoovered up the papadum crumbs.

On Sunday morning I raked up leaves in the garden and had a bonfire. It was a beautiful autumn day—dazzling sunshine and quite warm. As I planted pansies and spring bulbs in the pots and tubs, I came across dozens of nasturtium seeds that had fallen onto the gravel path. I collected them up and placed them in the borders, wondering if I would be there to see them flower next summer.

Then it was Tuesday, two days to go until I would have the results. My nice GP telephoned me to say she was going away for half term and had tried unsuccessfully to get my results from the hospital. She asked if I had enough support and told me I sounded very positive. All of these small kindnesses made a big difference. However, that was earlier in the day. Now I was frightened and for the first time, I felt sick with anxiety. I declined several offers from my friends to come with me to the hospital and decided that I certainly would not put my sister Jane through the ordeal as it was bound to stir up memories and emotions she would rather forget. I would go on my own. I made sure I had a nice weekend to look forward to, whatever the news. A good friend had invited me to Cornwall so I suggested that we meet up and arrange a meal with my cousin Anne and her husband, Robert, who live in Truro.

On Wednesday, Laura broke up for half term at lunchtime. I was determined not to let anything spoil our day as she and Alex were shortly leaving for their trip to France. We went to the Rockbourne Fair at Salisbury racecourse and enjoyed perusing the craft stalls and buying early Christmas presents. That evening I received a phone call from Jane who said she had decided to accompany me to the hospital the next day. That was good. Alex would be at a university open day and Laura was going to London with friends to see *The Sound of Music* so I would be able to process the news with some space before they returned.

By dawn on Thursday, I was wide awake. With a 2:30 p.m. appointment to be given my biopsy results, I needed to fill the morning so I arranged a routine visit to see a regular patient. I was pleased that my anxiety did not affect the horse, which responded positively to treatment and became profoundly relaxed, which in turn calmed me.

I arrived home at midday to find Jane waiting for me. We left plenty of time to make the twenty-minute journey to the hospital just in case there were any hold-ups. A cup of hot chocolate in the café passed another few minutes and then we made our way to surgical outpatients. Once we were called through from the general reception to the next waiting room, I became hyper-alert. I could not help but study the faces and demeanour of the other patients, who were quietly anxious. The room was full and crowded, with people arriving and being called through all the time. I remember the lady sitting next to me was reading *Country Life* magazine and the details of the article she was studying. As I sat there, waiting in suspense, I realised that the dice were already cast. *It is what it is*, I thought, and no amount of wishing or hoping would change the result now. In just a short while I would know.

I was taken into a small examination room and waited anxiously for the door to open. Miss Aertssen arrived, accompanied by one of the breast-care nurses, and introduced herself to Jane. She then kindly but matter-of-factly said that I had a ductal carcinoma in situ (DCIS) with no evidence of any spread on the samples examined. This was the best possible news under the circumstances and I felt a huge sense of relief. It meant that the cancer cells were confined to the ducts in the breast tissue and would not have spread to the rest of the breast or other parts of the body. As the tumour was four centimetres in diameter, she recommended a mastectomy which I would have requested anyway—anything to reduce the likelihood of spread or recurrence.

At the same time, they would remove a couple of lymph nodes for histology to be as certain as possible there was no spread elsewhere. I was offered a choice of dates: 27th November when Miss Aertssen returned from her holiday or a week earlier with one of her colleagues. Five weeks seemed a long time to wait and if given the choice, I would have had the operation much earlier, but as there was no perceived urgency, I chose to wait for Miss Aertssen to return as I liked and respected her. I knew it would make the operation less daunting if someone I had confidence in performed it.

Armed with yet more information leaflets and my own pink, breast-care file, I left the hospital in a celebratory mood. Jane stayed the night and we treated ourselves to a takeaway. I then had a lovely weekend in Cornwall with my friends. We took Anne and Robert out for an Indian meal on Saturday night and I kept my news to myself as I did not want it to cloud our precious time together. It was ironic that Anne shook her finger at me as we said our goodbyes and told me not to go getting any nasty diseases. She was thinking of my mother who was preparing to come to London for surgery, having been diagnosed with cancer for the third time. I decided not to tell them until I had the all-clear following surgery and there was no need to worry about me.

37

JUST WAITING

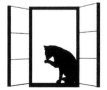

I n the intervening weeks, I kept busy with work and making preparations for my unexpected time off. One of the first things I had to do was to let Alex and Laura know what was happening in a way that would cause them minimal upset. I explained that the surgery should be curative and by Christmas, things would be more or less back to normal. In the meantime they would possibly have to give up a few of their activities as I would not be able to drive or lift anything for at least a couple of weeks. I was proud of them both at the way they handled the news. They were visibly upset but very brave for their mum.

It was a couple of weeks later that I began to feel that all was not well. Following the biopsies I had experienced minimal discomfort and relatively minor bruising. But now there were definite changes taking place. The next morning I telephoned the hospital for advice and was reassured that this sometimes happened and it was only two weeks until my surgery. However, from that moment on, the time could not pass fast enough for me. I was desperate to have the cancer removed from my body.

I filled my time with work, caring for the children and

attending more hospital appointments. I needed to do all my Christmas shopping and wrap up the presents. I even flew to Geneva to examine and treat an event horse belonging to the sister of one of my vet friends. It seemed amazing that I could leave home at lunchtime and by the following evening had been to Switzerland and back, made new friends and examined and treated a very special horse. The kindness of his owners touched me. We did not arrive at their home until nearly 11 p.m. and they had laid out a magnificent spread of different cheeses with fresh bread and an assortment of biscuits.

I felt quite a weight of responsibility as they had paid my airfare and car-parking fee and I had intended to go straight to bed and prepare for the next day's work. However, the conversation was stimulating; the kitchen was lovely and warm and we enjoyed the cheese and sipped red wine until retiring at 1 a.m. As I lay in bed, I marvelled at how relaxed and happy I felt. I slept well and woke up to bright sunshine and a crisp, chilly morning. The air was cold and pure; in the distance there was fresh snow on the mountains.

We drove to meet my patient, who was certainly worthy of all the efforts to make him comfortable. Gentle, friendly and beautifully behaved, this flea-bitten, grey gelding whinnied in welcome as we entered the barn. Time flew by as I examined and treated him and all too soon I was back at Geneva airport. I touched down at Gatwick at 7:30 p.m. and was back in Salisbury in time to have a few hours' sleep before the next hospital appointment.

* * *

When I look back through my diary, I am amazed at how positive and active I was leading up to my operation. For Alex and Laura, I tried to keep life as normal and happy as possible.

Each of us dealt with my diagnosis differently. Alex immediately confided in his friends, who were very supportive, whereas Laura refused to tell anyone. I informed the teachers at their respective schools where the information was treated with kindness and respect for each of their wishes. For my part I tried not to think about it any more than absolutely necessary. I continued to treat horses but as the date grew closer, I deferred taking on any new patients until the New Year. Without exception the owners were supportive and understanding, wishing me all the best.

Closer to home, support came in numerous ways. My next-door neighbour Charlie offered to do all the school runs, which I gratefully accepted, and my sister Jane gave me all sorts of tips for the time immediately after surgery. Little things such as taking pyjamas and cardigans that button up at the front rather than trying to pull anything over my head. Rosie gave me a beautiful, 500-piece jigsaw puzzle with three foals peering over a fence in case I was bored at home after the op. Then there were extensive pre-operative tests to check my blood count, my heart and medical history. I was swabbed for MRSA and thankfully that was all clear.

One day I escaped from my normal daily routine to meet my great friend Karen (another equine vet) at the Wildlife Photographer of the Year exhibition at the Natural History Museum. It was mid-November and the Christmas lights were already on. After losing ourselves in the amazing photographs, there was time for coffee and a chat before visiting hours at the London clinic where my mother was having complex cancer surgery. These outings helped the time pass before the all-important day.

Surgery was scheduled for 27th November and I did not book any work the day before. In the evening, Alex, Laura and I went into Salisbury to see the Christmas lights switched on in the market square. The atmosphere was very jolly with the late-night shoppers in festive mood, singing carols and chatting. By chance we met up with friends and watched the stunning firework display together. I enjoyed every moment, knowing that it was the last 'normal' time we would share for a while.

38

OPERATION DAY

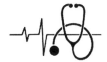

I had taken sleeping tablets for a few nights before the surgery to ensure I reached the day in the best possible shape. Insomnia has been a frequent companion since childhood, which is probably why I had always coped so well with being on call and instantly alert with every summons. I woke up bright and early in a cheerful mood but, uh-oh, I had a sore throat.

I debated whether I should mention it as I did not want anything to delay my surgery but then sensibly decided that the people responsible for my well-being—especially the anaesthetist—should know all the facts to be able to do their job optimally. I dressed in my favourite, comfy, blue FatFace outfit and asked Laura to photograph me in the kitchen, all ready to go.

What happened next will surely make the mothers of teenage boys smile. I needed to be in the surgical admissions lounge at 8 a.m. and always one for punctuality, asked Alex to take me there in his small car, ready to leave for the twenty-minute drive at 7:30 a.m. It was a frosty morning and he went out to start the car but reappeared a few minutes later to collect buckets of warm water to defrost the windscreen. Slightly anxious by this point, I then had to take a deep breath when he said, 'I don't think I dare risk warming the car with the engine on as the fuel indicator's on the low end of red. Could we stop at a garage on the way? I don't think there's enough petrol in the tank to reach the hospital.'

Although I was outwardly smiling but definitely worried, we managed to fill up his tank and still arrive just before 8 a.m. I waved him off for his day at school and walked into the now very familiar hospital where I was met by Izzy, who had taken the day off work and insisted that I should not go alone.

Shortly after our arrival, I was sent down to radiology in preparation for a sentinel node biopsy to determine if the cancer had spread. Two young doctors did the procedure with total professionalism and managed to make me smile. I felt in safe hands as I lay on my back experiencing mild discomfort as they injected the dye and manoeuvred the gigantic gamma cameras around me. After a short wait, the doctors made marks on my skin with a special marker pen to help the surgeon accurately locate the nodes and remove them with the minimum of trauma.

Then it was back up to the ward for a chat and yet another check-over by the anaesthetist. I confessed to having a sore throat but we agreed that the operation was a priority and should go ahead as I felt well.

* * *

Now it was time to go to theatre. I am sure Miss Aertssen came to see me but I cannot actually remember it. I have a fear of anaesthetics and worry that I will not wake up. The bit I hate most of all is the counting down and the bit I like most is waking up. This team were marvellous and spared me that anxiety. One moment I was engaged in conversation and the next thing I experienced was waking up in recovery. I had not noticed the anaesthetic being administered—perfect technique! As I regained consciousness, I thought about the procedure I had just had and asked myself how much it hurt. Lying there with my eyes shut, I felt remarkably comfortable. Feeling relaxed and sleepy, I was taken back to Downton Ward on a trolley and was able to wriggle over onto the bed. I remember looking at the clock and watching the minutes tick by.

I then lifted the blanket covering my chest, expecting to see bandages, but there was only a large, clear dressing through which the scar was visible. It was neat and unobtrusive, with a drain to collect any leakage from the wound. Shortly afterwards, Miss Aertssen appeared and told me the operation had gone well and that she would see me in the clinic in a week for the histology results. When I said I was surprised that there was so little discomfort, she advised me to wait until the local anaesthetic wore off, but it is a testament to her surgical skill that I remained much more comfortable than I had expected.

Later in the afternoon, Izzy came to see me, and Laura and Alex came up after school. They brought a nice card and pretty yellow roses—my favourite flowers. I chatted a little to the other patients and wrote my diary in the evening, before a restless night as the lady in the next bed snored like an express train. By Saturday morning I was more than ready to go home. It was chilly but sunny when Izzy collected me and wrapped her maroon shawl around my shoulders. Whenever possible we meet in Salisbury for coffee on a Saturday morning, so determined to keep things as normal as possible, we stopped in the market square and picked up take-away coffees from Costa, with a crème brûlée latte for me.

When we arrived home, I snuggled under a duvet on the pale grey leather settee in the conservatory with the cats for company and read a book before having a snooze. It was lovely to be home and even nicer to be looked after so well by Alex and

Laura in the days that followed. Alex would stop at Tesco on the way home from school and carry the bags of shopping on the bus. During the day I pottered around and did my stretching exercises, marking the place I could reach on the wall, right beside the children's height and date marks. The district nurse called a couple of times but I soon decided I was happy to dress my wound.

The days of the first week passed in a blurred memory of frequent visitors and wonderful cards and flowers. I photographed the flowers to provide a special memory of this time when everyone was so kind. I based myself in the conservatory, which is full of light and overlooks the garden. It has no heating but a couple of portable heaters kept me snug and warm. I remembered the good advice that my sister Jane gave me about limiting the number of visitors per day and the length of time they stay. I did get very tired answering the phone and eventually left a message on the answer phone thanking people for calling and saying that I was doing very well but could not chat at that moment.

On a couple of occasions, I became mildly concerned about the drain becoming blocked or localised swelling around the wound, but I only had to telephone the breast care department and no matter how busy they were, either Sonya or Shirley would reassure me or invite me in for a quick check. Each time I could see that they were not at all worried but they never made me feel as though I had been a nuisance. Every little kindness helped because whilst I was outwardly cheerful and thankful that everything had gone well so far, deep down I harboured an anxiety that would not abate until the histology results were back.

39

THE RESULTS

W hat happened next just goes to show that no amount of positive thinking can influence some outcomes. I had been brave, positive and probably in denial, determined that everything was going to be all right. I was still not allowed to drive, and Rosie kindly insisted on taking me to the follow-up appointment at the hospital.

She collected me at 2:30 p.m. for a 3:30 p.m. appointment. We sat in the bursting-to-the-seams waiting room, making conversation to fill the time, knowing that the information I was shortly to receive would influence the course of the next year and possibly the rest of my life. We were called into the examination room where Shirley removed my drain—an unpleasant but momentary experience. I was pleased to be free of the drainage bag with its pretty cover that had been hanging around my neck for the last week. Just a couple more days and the wound would be healed enough for me to soak in a warm bath again.

When Miss Aertssen arrived, we had a quick chat about how well I felt before she told me the histology results. After all those days and weeks of positive thinking on my part, she told me that the four-centimetre tumour contained several tiny foci of invasive cancer cells, the largest of which was two millimetres. This was too small for accurate grading but they did know that it did not have any oestrogen receptors. This meant that hormone therapy was not a treatment option so I would be offered chemotherapy and radiotherapy. The good news was that no invasion of the blood vessels was seen in the breast tissue and they were optimistic that all of the cancer had been removed. My lymph nodes were expected to be clear but the results would not be available for another week.

When she started saying all this, I suddenly felt distanced from Miss Aertssen who was standing by the examination couch, holding my notes in a folder. It was as though I had taken a step back and was looking in from the outside. As she delivered the news, my brain was questioning everything. Hang on a moment, this was not meant to happen. If you asked me to name my worst fears, being diagnosed with cancer and having chemotherapy would be close to the top. My usual chattiness deserted me and all I could say was, 'Oh.'

Stunned into quiet submission, I managed to ask when the chemotherapy would start and before I left the room a nurse handed me a piece of paper with my first oncology appointment in the Pembroke Suite. As we left the hospital, I felt subdued and asked Rosie to take me into Salisbury to get a coffee. There was still hope that the lymph nodes would be clear but realism now reigned and I sensibly put positive expectations on hold.

During the next week, I sometimes looked in the mirror and savoured the moments when I still looked like me. I dressed in pink and smiled at my reflection. I was still not driving and was delighted to receive a phone call from Jane, one of my very best friends from vet school. Her mum was treating her to a week of winter sunshine in Egypt and they would call in on their way from Devon to Gatwick. I knew her mum from my student days when we stayed with her in Wales and always enjoyed her company. Jane is one of those friends that I do not need to see often to maintain a close friendship. We had been through some difficult times together and are godmothers to each other's sons. Being perfect guests, they brought the lunch—a delicious macaroni cheese and salad. We sat in the warm conservatory and chatted companionably all afternoon. When Laura arrived home from school, she took a photo of us that to this day I treasure. I still have it propped up on the bookshelf in my office as a reminder of a special and happy afternoon.

For the rest of that week, life continued as normally as possible with Ella, an elderly black Labrador coming to stay whilst her owners went on holiday. I managed to attend Alex's parents' evening at school and Laura's carol service in Salisbury Cathedral. I said more than one little prayer for my family and me. And then it was Thursday again, time for another late-afternoon appointment at the hospital. This time I went on my own and had no optimistic expectations. Miss Aertssen confirmed that a very small number of cancer cells were present in the sentinel lymph node but the next lymph node was clear so hopefully it had all been surgically removed.

It was inevitable that during this time I began to wonder 'What if…?' Why had the lump reached four centimetres without me noticing? Would it have made any difference if the surgery had been sooner? These were just a couple of the questions that plagued my thoughts. Of course, this questioning was unproductive and unhelpful. I needed to deal with the situation as it was, rather than think about what might have been. In the end I turned my thinking around and focused on how *lucky* it was that I had thought to check myself that day, otherwise the cancer might still be growing and spreading undetected. Then maybe the delay allowed the small groups of cancer cells in the lymph node to develop sufficiently to be detected, rather than be present but not visible on the samples examined. I am not a histopathologist and my reasoning may be flawed, but it made me feel better.

Newspapers at the time devoted a considerable amount of space to debates on the effectiveness of breast screening and how breast cancer patients were often over-treated. The articles claimed that ladies with DCIS often underwent unnecessary mastectomies for non-invasive cancers that were never going to progress any further. So I would like to put the other side of the story because all three of the core biopsies indicated that my tumour was non-invasive and it was only after the whole breast was removed that the real picture emerged. If it had not been for the belt-and-braces thoroughness of the whole team at Salisbury District Hospital, I might not be telling my story today.

The important task now was to let Alex and Laura know what was in store. I ended up telling them individually as Laura had already broken up from school for the Christmas holidays and was at home when I got back. Both were outwardly exceptionally brave; I think it helped that they had seen their aunty Jane come through the treatment and make a good recovery. Whilst at the hospital, I had asked Miss Aertssen if it was OK for me to drive down to Devon the next day (I was going to go, whatever she said) and we planned a weekend of fun and family time to deflect our thoughts from the treatment to come.

40

MY LOVE OF DONKEYS

When you receive a cancer diagnosis, it tends to stop you in your tracks. Silly things that were previously irritating fall into perspective as you suddenly see the bigger picture. My senses and appreciation of all the good things were heightened: the colours of falling leaves, the fragrance of fresh flowers and the warmth of a log fire. Then there was beautiful music that seemed especially poignant.

Something I had always wanted to do was attend the candlelight carol service at the Donkey Sanctuary in Devon. It was that time of year so Laura and I set off in the wintry sunshine the very next day, with Laura grumbling most of the way. Even pancakes and maple syrup at a Little Chef en route failed to sweeten her mood as we headed southwest. The special atmosphere of the Donkey Sanctuary at Sidmouth soon changed all that. We arrived just as the sun set and the sky was a vivid pink and deepening blue. The chill hit us as we left the warmth of the car and headed down into the main visitors' yard. And there to our delight was Jubilee, the elderly donkey who had come to live with us for a while as a companion to Joan, our own donkey. Of the 3,000 donkeys at the sanctuary, Jubilee had been selected for the nativity scene. He looked happy and well, as always enjoying being the centre of attention.

After making a big fuss of Jubilee and answering some of the other visitors' questions about him, we headed towards the mulled wine and mince pies, which helped to warm us up. By now the sanctuary was filling with people from far and wide. All had come to see the donkeys and support the work done to improve the welfare of donkeys and mules worldwide. That evening, over 15,000 candles were lit, each one with a £1 donation in memory of a loved friend, relative or pet or with good wishes for someone in need. The written messages were in a giant tub under a decorated tree and the burning candles lined the pathways. In the indoor school used to give therapy to children with special needs and disabilities, candles were arranged in the shape of stars, angels, Christmas trees and snowmen. The scene was enchanting and magical, with donkeys in the background contentedly munching on hay and straw.

As the band warmed up, our fingers and toes went numb in the freezing cold. We gathered in the main yard for the 45-minute carol service. 'O Come, All Ye Faithful' and 'Silent Night' were spiritual, whilst the 'Calypso Carol' was joyful and celebratory. I stepped back from the crowd and leant on the railings, becoming momentarily detached, thinking about the course of my life and how much I still hoped to do. My retirement plan has always been to help the Donkey Sanctuary with their overseas programmes, setting up clinics and helping the people who depend on donkeys and mules for their livelihood to look after them better. Donkeys have always had a special place in my heart. When Joan came to live with us as a companion for my horse, she brought an aura of gentleness and peace to our home.

Laura came and snuggled up to me for warmth and we watched a Jack Russell puppy playing in the straw. Then the band started to play 'Little Donkey' and it all became just too poignant, as Joan had passed away the previous year. I was not the only one with silent tears and treasured memories that evening.

With the service over and our prayers said, we jumped into the car with the heaters on full blast and made our way to spend the evening with Alex, the senior vet at the sanctuary, her partner, Bob, and their three delightful children. Over a meal of chilli con carne, we caught up with the news and wondered where the years had gone. Alex and I had worked as young vets in Salisbury and now here we were with teenage children of our own. It was a companionable time that balanced my emotional moments earlier on. I was very touched to be given two gifts to help me through the forthcoming chemotherapy: a beaded, good-luck necklace from Gambia and a book of meaningful quotations entitled *Walk Beside Me and Be My Friend*, produced by the animal welfare charity SPANA (Society for the Protection of Animals Abroad). Each quotation was accompanied by a photograph of donkeys at work, rest and play from around the world.

The next morning Laura and I collected my son, Alex, from Exeter station and went on to Ilfracombe to spend the day with and deliver Christmas presents to my aunty Beryl and cousin Christopher in Ilfracombe. Another day of happy chatting, reminiscing and family time before the long drive home to chill out in front of a log fire with Saturday evening TV.

41

PREPARING FOR CHEMOTHERAPY

We were now well into December and I decided to wait until January to start the treatment. It was all such unknown territory and it was important to me that this Christmas was special and not spoilt by feeling unwell.

I also wanted to give my body time to recover. The area around my scar was initially numb but then became ultra-sensitive to even the light touch of loose clothing. I experimented with various dressings and discovered that if I wore a close-fitting crop top, it protected my skin from this irritation that went away after a few weeks.

The preparation for receiving the treatment was exceptionally thorough. My first appointment was with Belinda, the chemotherapy nurse practitioner. It was with trepidation that I located the Pembroke Suite where treatment is carried out. It was in the older part of the hospital, next door to the Beatrice Wards where I had given birth to my children. I took a deep breath and opened the door to the unit that would be an important feature of the next six months. On first impressions it was bright and scrupulously clean. I checked in at reception and went to the empty waiting room. There was a fridge full of water and soft drinks; on the low tables were piles of the latest women's magazines. A male cleaner worked quietly, moving every chair and leaving no nook or cranny untouched.

Belinda collected me and took me to an examination room. She went through an extensive questionnaire and allowed me to discuss any concerns or queries. She gave me a personal diary that contained information on all aspects of chemotherapy, including the emergency contact telephone numbers to call if I was worried at any time. I remember no stone being left unturned with regard to my health and welfare. We discussed the side effects and how to minimise them, although this was an unknown quantity as people have very individual responses to the cytotoxic chemotherapy. The drugs target fast-growing cancer cells but also affect healthy cells that multiply quickly so the symptoms tend to reflect disturbances to cells of the bone marrow, digestive tract and reproductive system as well as the skin and hair follicles.

In my mind I had a stereotypical image of chemotherapy patients as frail and thin, feeling nauseous and losing their hair. I was soon to learn how false and narrow this picture was. Since I was desperate to do anything to increase my chances of survival, I enquired about special diets and nutritional supplements. Anything I forgot to ask Belinda or needed reassurance with was addressed when I met Dr Crowley, my oncology consultant, three days later. I'm not sure what I expected her to look like but she was younger and prettier than I had imagined. More importantly, she was kind and caring, which made me feel comfortable.

Away from the hospital, there was a lot to organise. I needed an urgent dental check-up to ensure my mouth was free of infection or other potential problems. I was vaccinated against various types of flu and pneumonia. I made an appointment to see Jane, my GP, who was very supportive and always at the end of the phone if I had any worries.

The chemotherapy nurses had suggested that there was no point in having any more highlights in my hair as it was likely to fall out anyway but Barbara, my very good friend and hairdresser, had other ideas. We agreed that it was important to look and feel good for Christmas and went ahead as planned. I wanted a single, pink streak in my fringe as a declaration of my determination to survive breast cancer but there she drew the line and suggested that if I must, I could buy a clip-on extension at Claire's Accessories.

The big unknown that worried me most was 'How sick was I going to be?' Would I be able to cook, shop, run the house, care for the children and work? It is at times like this that as a single parent with no family nearby, you feel very alone. My mother would be undergoing chemotherapy with her schedule a month or so behind mine. My sisters and friends had families and responsibilities of their own. But then out of the blue, I had a phone call from my cousin Anne, offering to come up from Cornwall and stay with me for a few days each time I received treatment. It was the perfect solution as I would be relaxed in her company and not feel that I had to pretend to feel fine even when I didn't. She said however horrid I was, she would not go away. Thank you, Anne.

By now the Christmas festivities were underway and at a drinks party in the village I received countless good wishes and offers of support, which I knew were genuine. Once the New Year had arrived, I would be ready. But for now I was going to make sure this was the best Christmas ever.

CHRISTMAS 2009

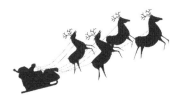

My favourite day of the year has always been Christmas Eve. I love the fairy lights, tinsel and festive carols and the fun of wrapping up the presents that I have carefully selected. That year I had a wonderful day. Alex, Laura and I went into Salisbury to meet Izzy and her daughters, Katie and Megan. We exchanged presents over mugs of steaming hot chocolate and sticky treats at a café, then the young people left us to wander around town, leaving Izzy and me to chat. We have been friends since meeting in the maternity ward at Salisbury District Hospital eighteen years previously. Katie was born three days before Alex and Laura is four months older than Meg. It became a tradition that we shared a tea party in September each year to celebrate the older children's birthdays. As they grew up, the jelly and chocolate caterpillar cake were replaced by evening visits to Italian restaurants and we have photos of every year from one to eighteen as treasured reminders.

After the hustle and bustle of the build-up for Christmas, Salisbury is often quiet on Christmas Eve. We wandered amongst the stalls in the market square, buying fresh Brussels sprouts and spontaneous, last-minute extras. Then it was home to peel vegetables and prepare the turkey. On the back doorstep, I found an arrangement of white flowers from my mother and a package with Jo Malone body lotion from one of her friends— such special and thoughtful surprises.

Another of our Christmas traditions is drinking mulled wine and enjoying mince pies with our neighbours. When I moved into the village of Farley in 1987, it was lovely to be welcomed into the community. The residents included a whole range of professional people and local craftsmen. However, the one thing that I missed was having a special friend and then when I was expecting Alex, I realised that there were no other young children in the village. Imagine my delight when Eileen, a doctor, and her husband, Michael, moved in with their baby son, Paul. The boys grew up together—completely different in character but firm friends. The gang of two became four when Paul's brother, Charles, was born three months before Laura.

Until this particular year, we had always attended the 3 p.m. crib service at Farley Church together and then gathered at Eileen's house afterwards for mulled wine. Now the youngsters declared themselves too old for a crib service so we met up mid-afternoon. As a surprise Michael had cooked a delicious lasagne and this was followed by Eileen's apple crumble. Afterwards we exchanged secret Santa presents and particularly enjoyed the occasion as the boys and Laura had selected the presents for each other for the first time and it was interesting to see their choices: a guitar tuner for Charles, candles for Laura and beers for the older boys. Then it was time to come home as our friends headed to Salisbury Cathedral for midnight mass.

With Alex and Laura in bed, I listened to carols on the television as I performed my Father Christmas duties. To this day he still leaves footprints of ash on the hearthrug and a nibbled carrot because the reindeer are too full from their previous visits to finish it. I leave out a chilled Diet Coke instead of an alcoholic beverage; it is a joke we have enjoyed for some years.

As I completed my task at 1 a.m. in front of the fire's glowing embers and the twinkling tree lights, I felt that everything was very special and nothing could be nicer. Christmas Day followed in the same spirit and then whilst Alex went to a party, Laura and I saw in the New Year together, wondering just what 2010 had in store for us.

43

THE NEW YEAR

O n reflection it is usually possible to find some unexpected and positive aspects to difficult times. As I sat in my warm conservatory, watching from the comfort of my settee as the garden birds hungrily ate the seeds and nuts, it occurred to me that if this had to happen, then now was the best time of year. It was the quietest period for my work and I was not missing being outside in the cold weather as I often struggled to keep warm in the winter.

It was also a cosy time for the children and me when we just got on and managed everything between us. To their delight I bought a second TV in the sales after Christmas and had Sky multi-room installed, recognising that I would probably watch it more than usual and did not want to share their viewing of *The Simpsons*, rugby or teen soaps.

I noticed too that since the operation, I had not needed to visit the chiropractor and my feet no longer hurt. My body was getting a rest from the long hours in the car and the physical demands of continually examining and treating horses, but by the first week of January, I felt fit and was more than ready to start work again. On Monday morning I was delighted to go and see Lucky, a very cheeky horse I had treated for many years. It felt so good to be back and I found I could move and stretch as normal, with no restrictions from the scar tissue. Treating Lucky and chatting to his owner reassured me that I was indeed fully recovered.

I had a busy week planned with visits to a racing stable, an eventing yard and to see a couple of other favourite patients before the chemotherapy started the following Monday. However, it was not to be. This was a week of heavy snowfalls and by Wednesday, our village was almost completely cut off from the outside world. Schools closed; the buses could not get through and the roads were barely passable with four-wheel-drive vehicles and then only with care. Laura stayed at home and we enjoyed some lovely walks in the woods, which were like a winter wonderland. With my heightened sense of appreciation and imagination, I felt as though I had stepped into the land of Narnia. Alex was not so lucky as he had been unable to get home from school on Wednesday evening and was staying with friends in Salisbury.

Luckily I had had my final pre-treatment appointment at the hospital on the Tuesday afternoon. The chemotherapy nurses confirmed that I would have a Groshong line put in on Friday morning. This is a permanent catheter tunnelled under the skin with a fine, silicone tube inserted into a large vein leading directly to the heart. It meant that the intravenous drugs could be given via this line and it removed the need to keep using veins in my hands and arms. I opted for this because my sister warned me that one of the worst problems was the soreness of her arms from frequent intravenous injections with the irritant drugs.

By Thursday evening I knew that I needed to accept one of the many offers of help from friends in the village. The road outside my driveway has quite a steep slope and was still a no-go area for ordinary cars such as mine. And so it was that Jill and Jamie turned up on Friday morning to take me to the hospital in their Land Rover. We drove slowly along the narrow country lanes with snow piled high on each side and then were amazed to find almost no snow at all in Salisbury.

I felt nervous as I checked in at the radiology department and after the procedure was explained, I accepted the offer of sedation, reckoning it would make it easier for everyone. Lying on my back on the radiography table, surrounded by the ultrasound and X-ray equipment used to locate the vein and check the placement of the catheter, I was surprised at the size of the team involved. Sarah, the nurse, sat close to my head, monitoring my vital signs and administering oxygen. There were two scrub nurses (one was training the other) preparing me for the sterile procedure, two radiographers, three doctors (two learning) and a student. The last thing I remember was being covered with a large green drape and being given the sedative, then I slept through the entire procedure. When I woke up, I was taken for an X-ray to check the position of the catheter and then up to the Pembroke Suite to recover.

This was the first time I'd been in the treatment area of the unit and it was not in the least bit how I'd imagined it would be. It was bright and airy with an upbeat, positive atmosphere, smiley faces and a background sound of friendly banter. The nurses on the unit settled me into a bed and took some blood so they had the figures as a reference starting point and could monitor my red and white cell count, platelets and liver and kidney function as treatment proceeded. A nurse showed me how to change the dressing over my Groshong line and once I was fully awake, I sat in a comfortable chair and chatted to some of the other patients. Then Anne, one of the nurses, made my day by telling me that the book I had written on the veterinary care of the horse was the favourite one in her collection. That really bucked my spirits up and helped me feel as though I was part of this whole scene rather than the new girl on the ward.

Jamie later collected me and I went home determined to make the most of and enjoy every minute of the forthcoming weekend with the children.

44

INTO THE UNKNOWN

My first chemotherapy was scheduled for 9 a.m. on Monday 11th January 2010. My cousin Anne had arrived the previous afternoon and once the children had left for school, I could not stand waiting around for a minute longer, so we set off for the hospital with a stop at the supermarket on the way. I was feeling very anxious about the as yet unknown effect that the treatment would have on me. At the top of the shopping list was a washing-up bowl to go by my bed, just in case.

We need not have hurried. I quickly learnt to put aside the whole day as there was often a delay of one sort or another. My assigned nurse for this session was Maggs, who was friendly, efficient and cheerful. I was given the choice of sitting on a bed or a comfy chair and unless other patients needed them, I always chose a bed. The first task for Maggs was to flush my Groshong line with saline. The nurses then attached me to a saline drip whilst they ordered and checked the chemotherapy drugs. Next, I was given a small pot containing a number of little white pills to swallow, a mixture of corticosteroids and anti-emetic drugs to stop me feeling sick from the treatment.

My treatment was known as FEC chemotherapy, which combined the drugs' initials: fluorouracil (5FU), epirubicin and cyclophosphamide. I was to have six chemotherapy sessions at three-week intervals. As the drugs are so toxic, the nurses wore gloves and aprons to protect them from any accidental contact. Before anything was administered, the assigned nurse brought over a colleague and the name of the drug, the dose, its expiry date and the name, hospital number and date of birth of the patient were called out. Once they were checked, the nurse injected the clear, bright pink epirubicin very slowly over several minutes into a port on the drip tube. This was a good opportunity for me to get to know the nurse and discuss any early treatment concerns. A bag containing cyclophosphamide was then attached to the drip and once this had finished and been flushed through with saline, I was given the 5FU. Apart from feeling anxious as the drugs ran in, the only sensation I had was a tingling of my nose as the nurse administered cyclophosphamide.

During the treatment I was free to walk around the ward, make a cup of tea or visit the loo. I just took the drip stand with me. I had been warned that my wee would be bright pink so that was no surprise but looking in the mirror was. The face looking back at me was so white and pale with red-rimmed eyes. I was pleased that Anne had taken a photo of me attached to the drip and looking cheerful and healthy shortly after our arrival at the hospital.

I had brought a newspaper and a book with me but I spent most of that first treatment session looking around the ward observing the nurses, the other patients and the general activity going on around me. I could not help but wonder why each person was there. Most of them were my age or older and they all seemed very dignified and accepting of their situation. Some snoozed; others read magazines and a number brought a friend or partner along for company.

The side-effects are different for everyone but can include lowered resistance to infection, bruising or bleeding, anaemia, tiredness, hair loss, sore mouth and ulcers. Other possible symptoms are loss of taste or a metallic taste in your mouth, skin and nail changes, diarrhoea, constipation, sore eyes and bladder irritation. You are particularly vulnerable to infection seven to ten days after treatment when the white blood cells are at their lowest due to suppression of the bone marrow which produces red and white blood cells and platelets. During the morning a lady came into the ward for a blood transfusion as her platelets, which help the blood to clot, were very low and she was covered in bruises.

By early afternoon the treatment had finished. The nurses flushed my line again and gave me a bag of dressings and sterile wipes to keep it clean until my next appointment. Another bag contained everything necessary to flush the line myself at weekly intervals and the nurse went through the tablets that I would need to take for the next four days. It was very important to check that any other prescribed or self-administered medicines were compatible with the chemotherapy drugs. Finally, the nurses gave me an appointment for three weeks' time to have my next blood test and see the consultant. If all was well, then I would have the second treatment a day later.

When I was told I was free to go home, I was unsure what I should do. Go to bed? Sit quietly? Maggs said just to take it easy and see how I felt. She stressed that if I felt worried or unwell, I should telephone the Pembroke Ward emergency number, which is answered 24 hours a day. Back at home it felt most peculiar sitting and waiting for something unpleasant to happen. Anne and I waited…and waited…and I felt absolutely fine.

That night I did not sleep very well and eventually gave up and decided to read a book at 4 a.m. This was something I was going to get used to, along with feeling very hot at night. The next day I took it easy and felt completely normal. The tablets I was taking to stop me feeling sick worked perfectly; the only challenge was remembering which medication to take and when. By the third day, I was experiencing mild gastritis and constipation so the doctors added more pills and potions. I soon found it necessary to make a chart and tick off the various tablets as I swallowed them. I was pleased when they were all finished by Friday.

In the early stages of treatment, I decided to try and have an organic, dairy-free diet as some people believe this helps reduce the risk of developing breast cancer and has a positive effect on helping the body rid itself of the disease. This made the routine Tesco shop take three times as long as I had to read all the labels and discover previously unexplored areas of the store. I think I lasted a week before succumbing to some chocolate and deciding that I would simply make an effort to eat healthily instead. The compromise was to buy organic fruit and vegetables when possible but otherwise to enjoy my usual food. I was incredibly fortunate in not experiencing nausea throughout the entire treatment period. By the end I was half a stone (and a roll of fat around my tummy) heavier but that was distinctly preferable to feeing poorly. The weight gain I am sure was due to a combination of exercising less, taking corticosteroids for a few days after each treatment and simply not having the energy or willpower to watch my diet as carefully as normal.

Over the next few days, I was touched by the kindness of my friends and family but also people I did not know very well. The teachers at Alex and Laura's schools kept in contact and were always willing to help in any way. When I asked Laura's housemistress how much notice she would need for Laura to stay the occasional night at school if necessary, she said, 'Five minutes would be good but if I just find her in the dormitory that is also fine.' All in all I felt well cared for by the wider community and it gave me great comfort.

By Thursday I decided that I was probably well enough to work but I would take Anne with me in case I felt ill. It would have been nice to test myself with an easy horse near to home but life does not work like that. The three-day-event horses were now getting fit for the coming season so we set off for a yard 60 miles away to treat a gentle gelding and a very feisty one. I had also decided not to take on any new patients at this time and had to smile when I heard myself agree to treat a new horse that was not fond of needles.

The day went well. As soon as I was with the horses, any doubts I had about my health went away and my confidence returned. It was a wonderful and reassuring feeling as being able to work gave me a focus and sense of normality that helped me through the next few months. Without exception my clients were understanding and supportive. They gave me coffee, tea, sandwiches and chocolate in warm kitchens and tack rooms and a rest between horses if necessary. Poor Anne endured a long, cold day but having her there in those first days was a sensible precaution and made me feel safe.

All chemotherapy patients have to carry a card with them stating that they are undergoing treatment and listing emergency contact numbers in case they become unwell or are involved in an accident. As being kicked by a steel-clad hoof is a hazard of my job, I sellotaped an envelope to the dashboard of my car, clearly labelled 'In case of emergency', just in case I was injured or became unwell in the course of my work. Removing and ripping it up months later gave me great satisfaction.

Anne went home on Friday and Alex had a maths exam that was part of his A level. Several months earlier I had booked tickets for us to see Michael Morpurgo's *War Horse* in London on the Saturday with a group of friends. I took care not to sit near anyone with a cold on the train journey and we had a lovely evening with supper in a Covent Garden bistro before the performance. The choreography with the life-size horse puppets was so outstanding that I felt as though I was witnessing real horses on stage with every flick of an ear, mane or tail. Altogether it was a wonderful evening which showed that I was able to carry on as normal at present.

A week after the treatment, I went back to the hospital for a wig fitting—all part of the wonderful service from our NHS and a nice lady called Amanda. The first one that I picked out looked as though I was wearing a bush on my head. The second matched my own hair perfectly—highlights too—and fitted like a glove. I felt very fortunate and delighted that the wig looked natural and was comfortable. It made the thought of losing my hair more bearable. Then I went to meet Sarah in the psychology department to see if she could help with my sleep problem, which was getting worse. She warned me that I could be on a losing wicket as many chemotherapy patients who normally sleep well experience difficulty sleeping whilst receiving treatment. In the weeks ahead, Sarah helped me to look at my life in a way that would have a benefit lasting far longer than the duration of my cancer treatment. I realised that some of the things I was striving for in life were unrealistic goals and understanding this reduced my general anxiety levels.

In these early days, I had more time to myself and it was immensely satisfying to tackle and finish many jobs that had been waiting for a long time. My friends came to visit and we booked up treats to look forward to in the months ahead. Although I did feel tired some days, on the whole I was so relieved to feel well that it energised me to the extent that one night when I met Rosie in Prezzo's for supper, she told me that I looked more alive and pretty than she'd ever seen me and was probably the only person to have chemotherapy as a tonic.

Of course, it did not last…

45

LOOKING IN THE MIRROR

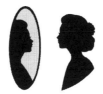

I do not consider myself to be a vain person but by the end of the second week, I could see some unwelcome changes in the mirror. I felt all right but the face that stared back at me was more lined than usual with red-rimmed eyes sunk in dark hollows.

The day inevitably came when my hair began to fall out. It was exactly two weeks after the first treatment and I was driving towards Winchester, on my way to see some favourite clients. As had become my habit, I gave my hair a little tug to check that it was still firmly rooted and out came a bunch of about twenty hairs. I consoled myself with the thought that at least the treatment was working.

When I arrived at the yard, I was greeted with a comforting hug. I was told that I was definitely needed to treat the horses throughout the year, which boosted my fragile morale. It was still January and although the sun was shining, the weather was cold and I noticed I was finding it increasingly difficult to keep warm. In between treating each horse, I was ushered into the tack room where I sat in front of an electric fire with a warm drink. This kindness and the three lovely horses turned the initially traumatic day into a very good one.

A couple of days later, I noticed that I left a trail of hair behind me wherever I went: on my pillow, in the hairbrush and just falling off my head in front of my eyes. I felt permanently cold and the lines seemed to be etched ever more deeply into my now thinner and older face. Between Thursday and Sunday, most of my hair fell out. Had I been grooming a horse, the feeling would have been very satisfying but with large tufts easily plucked from my head, it just felt sad. On Sunday morning I leant over the bath, running my fingers through my hair with the shower turned on, and watched it accumulate in the plughole. It was like saying goodbye to a friend.

Of course I knew this was going to happen and had taken some photos of me with the children and our new puppy a few days previously.

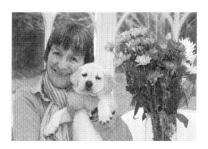

Then day by day, Laura took close-up shots and we loaded them onto my computer and made them into a slideshow. I was looking at my list of downloaded songs for some suitable music to go with them when I saw something that made me grin from ear to ear. Bryn Terfel singing 'Cavatina', with the words 'She Was Beautiful' became the accompaniment to my emerging baldness and to this day the song never ceases to make me smile.

Since I came to Salisbury in 1986, seeing Barbara, my

hairdresser, for a cut and blow dry has been a monthly treat. She did the highlights that were always a talking point with my younger clients who told me I was cool and refused to believe my real age, but more than that she has been a real friend. We have giggled like schoolgirls, shared confidences and even shed tears together with the ups and downs of our lives. She very kindly found me a second wig with wilder locks for those days when I felt like a change of style. In April she trimmed away the few straggling hairs that remained, so one way and another we still found excuses to keep in touch and enjoy a cup of coffee together.

As for the rest of my hair, well that all fell out too except for on my legs where it grew as fast as ever. How unfair was that? All in all the hair loss experience was not a good one but nowhere near as traumatic as I had feared.

HAVING A PUPPY

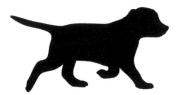

I have been lucky enough to own two special golden retrievers; the first was Honey and the second was CC. I was at a bar-b-q in Farley one summer evening several years ago when the topic of conversation turned to dogs. Most of my friends remembered the days when three Cavalier King Charles spaniels and Honey accompanied me to work, taking over all the available space in the car. When asked if I would consider having another dog, I replied that I would like a golden retriever but was not actively looking as I felt that one would find me when the time was right.

And sure enough, amongst the guests who heard my response was a lady who walked a lovely golden retriever belonging to two doctors. They had recently been promoted to consultant status and spent long hours at the hospital so were beginning to question whether it was fair to keep a dog and had considered the possibility of rehoming her. What happened next was inevitable. CC came for an introductory meeting and was so sweet and loveable that we immediately welcomed her into our family. I belatedly remembered that we were going camping at the weekend, but she was completely unfazed and just snuggled into the only available floor space between the children in the tent and made herself at home.

CC was eight years old at the time and we were lucky enough to share another seven years of unconditional love and companionship. I could take her anywhere and implicitly trust her in any situation; she just loved people. If the postman accidentally left the garden gate open, CC would head to the church, the pub or the village school. Our phone number was on her collar and one day a lady telephoned to say she was bringing her back from a children's party. CC had wandered up the road and gone in through the open front door where she enjoyed the games, shared the food and loved being petted by the youngsters. We had not yet realised she was missing.

When the time came to say goodbye in the summer of 2008, we buried her in the rose garden, where she had loved to bask in the sun, and planted some flowers in her memory. She had lost a lot of weight and although the time was right and the end was very peaceful, she left a huge gap that was waiting to be filled.

Alex and Laura were very keen on having a puppy and promised to do their share of training and caring for it. I had resisted for eighteen months as I felt life was too busy but when I received my cancer diagnosis, it occurred to me that it would be lovely to cuddle up with a puppy and the unexpected time at home would be ideal for house and obedience training. I had a vision of being snuggled up on the sofa with a sweet little girl puppy on my lap. I wanted another golden retriever but thinking of the muddy conditions in which I live and work, decided that it would be more sensible to have a short-coated Labrador. At the same time, common sense also nudged my conscience and reminded me that clearing up after a puppy was probably not ideal for an immunosuppressed chemotherapy patient.

Sometimes you knowingly make a questionable decision and hope for the best. And so it was that Rosie and I set off to collect Rafiki (which means 'friend' in Swahili), just before my second chemotherapy cycle. The pale yellow puppy was fast asleep on a low windowsill when we arrived to collect her. I wanted to try and make her first experience in the car a good one so when all the formalities were dealt with, I settled her on a comfy, fluffy towel on my lap for the journey home. She wriggled continuously and after ten minutes seemed distressed, panting and whining, so I transferred her to an open cardboard box with a cuddly Andrex puppy toy and a piece of Vetbed that smelled of her litter mates. It was not long before she started to yelp so we pulled over and thinking she might prefer the security of a large and enclosed cat travel box, we put her in there and set off again. We could only stand the subsequent howling for a short time and had to stop again. This time we let her explore the car and she settled down on Rosie's coat and slept happily all the way home.

When we got back, she gambolled around the garden and then investigated our utility room and kitchen. So full of fun, it was lovely to watch. In the evening she sat and played with us whilst we watched TV and then she went to bed in her dog box with the Andrex puppy, where she fell fast asleep without even a whimper.

However, this is a cautionary tale and I should probably have followed my instincts: if in doubt—don't. Although she was a wonderfully good-natured puppy, Rafiki was unlucky enough to have a couple of health issues that made her difficult to house train and ultimately put my health at risk. More of that later. Because she was not completely well, I had to delay vaccinating and socialising her and this caused me quite a bit of stress when I should have been concentrating on looking after myself. In my experience, vets often worry just as much or even more even more than most people when their pets are ill, especially if they do not recover as quickly as expected.

Now I have to dispel the image of a cuddly puppy sitting on my lap. How foolish was that! This did not happen until she was a solid 25-kilogram young adult when I would have preferred her at my feet. As a puppy, Rafiki never seemed to sit still and my lap was merely a springboard to the chest of drawers behind the chair, from which she would knock down all our ornaments and framed photos. No surface was safe; she could empty it with a sweep of her head or swipe of the tail and also elongate her length to reach even the middle of the kitchen table. In short, our house was trashed. I often thought that Tornado would have been a better name.

Recycling took on a new meaning as almost everything was chewed up and passed right though her. On a number occasions when clearing the garden, I was horrified to spy something that could so easily have caused a blockage in her gut and needed surgery to remove it. There was also the matter of her inexhaustible energy, which rated high on even the Labrador scale. Two of my friends in the village had black Labs the same age and it was a delight to watch them all play together. The other two then slept on their beds for the rest of the day, whereas Rafiki ran to fetch her ball the minute we arrived home.

As she approached her first birthday, I could genuinely say that I loved my dog and was pleased we bought her, but would I recommend anyone in my situation do the same? Definitely not.

A ROCKY ROAD

At the beginning of February, I was given my second chemotherapy treatment by Jill, one of my favourite nurses. The blood test showed that my white cell count was down a bit, but nothing to worry about. I did, however, have problems with my Groshong line, which was still discharging a little around the exit site from my chest and needed daily cleaning and dressing. I had naively assumed that the line would be a trouble-free part of me for the five months and would have no disadvantages whatsoever. This was not the case.

The chemotherapy was administered without a hitch then cousin Anne, who again came up from Truro to look after me, drove us home and cooked toad in the hole for supper. This delighted the children as a nice change from our usual, predictable menus. The next day she went home as she felt a cold coming on and did not want to give it to me. I felt a bit tired and irritable after the treatment but watching Sky Sports and seeing some racehorses that I had recently treated running at the Meydan Racecourse in Dubai cheered me up. By Sunday I was shivering with a temperature and a streaming cold and found it a difficult and lonely day as the children were spending the weekend with their father. I gave up fighting the virus and slept on the settee in the conservatory. At the same time, poor Rafiki was troubled with cystitis-like symptoms that led to the demise of the lounge carpet. It was a miserable time.

The next day was Laura's birthday but I did not see her in the morning as she went to school from her dad's house. Most of the day I stayed in bed still feeling rough, but I managed to get up briefly to wrap her presents. Eileen and Michael very kindly did an impromptu birthday party for her in the evening with a delicious feast of roast chicken followed by chocolate brownies. This made the day special in a way that I could not have done myself and was one of the many occasions when I appreciated the thoughtfulness and generosity of my friends.

It was not long before I recovered and it was wonderful to feel well again. Life got back to normal and I was busy at work. Rafiki was now much more comfortable and loved coming with me, travelling well in the boot of the car and quite happy to be tied up in the stable yards with a comfy bed. I would often have a quick break between patients and take her for a little walk. The not-so-good news was that the novelty of owning a puppy wore off very quickly for my teenagers who relinquished their share of her care with one excuse or another.

My third chemotherapy was planned for Monday 22nd February, coinciding with Take Your Child to Work Day at Laura's school. She decided that visiting the Pembroke Suite and watching me have treatment would be more interesting than another day watching me work as she had often accompanied me during the school holidays when she was younger. We planned her visit and both the nurses and her teachers were happy to accommodate this and thought it might help her to understand what was happening to her mum. I suggested to Anne that she did not come up from Cornwall this time as I had not experienced any side-effects after either of the first two treatments. She very kindly offered to be on standby instead.

The waiting room at the hospital was packed so we had to wait a while for my blood test and then go for a cup of coffee whilst it was analysed. Unfortunately this time I had very low total white cell and granulocyte counts as the treatment had suppressed my bone marrow, meaning that I was particularly vulnerable to infection. Belinda, the chemotherapy nurse practitioner, gave me the option of delaying the treatment or going ahead and having injections to stimulate my bone marrow on days five to ten of this and each subsequent treatment cycle. I chose the latter and continued as planned. Laura was good company and Belinda was very kind and answered all her questions. It was a long day as I also had an ECG because my heart was beating erratically when I lay in certain positions due to irritation from the tip of my Groshong line.

At the end of the day, I felt incredibly tired. Rosie and I had arranged to meet at the local pub for a meal to celebrate being halfway through the treatment. In reality, halfway is just before the fourth treatment rather than just after the third and as I was about to find out, a lot can happen in that time. Having supper out was not a good idea. I felt decidedly jaded and shortly after we started our meal, an elderly couple with heavy colds came and sat at the adjacent table. We promptly moved to the other bar and continued our meal there.

Two days later I discovered the meaning of the word fatigue. Whilst pushing the trolley through the supermarket, I was suddenly overcome with an overwhelming tiredness. I can remember seeing a big empty space on the bottom shelf in the cereal section and wanting to crawl into it and fall asleep. I would not have minded or noticed the other shoppers' reactions as I was past caring and could barely make it to the checkout. There were other jobs on my list, but I had to abandon those and have a rest because later in the afternoon I had an appointment for Rafiki to see a small animal vet. The previous day she had passed some blood when straining to go to the toilet and had whimpered with the effort so I had dropped a faecal sample off at the lab. Sam, the vet, told me that she had a protozoal parasite that did not usually cause any symptoms but she would like to cast an eye over my puppy whilst waiting for further results from the bacteriology lab. Although Rafiki was bright and happy, she did have a tender abdomen and needed to start some medication.

The next day began well but soon started to go downhill. I had had a good night's sleep and felt much better. I was on my way to treat some horses with Rafiki in the boot of my car when I had a phone call from Sam to say that *Campylobacter* had been grown from her faecal samples. Help! This is a bacterium that can cause serious diarrhoea in humans and other animals, so I could not possibly continue my journey to see clients with a puppy that was a potential public health risk. At first, I headed for home but then realised I was not happy to leave Rafiki all day on her own. I also needed to find out what the implications were for me with my reduced immunity.

I phoned Sam back and accepted her kind offer of hospitalising my pup in the isolation kennels. Rafiki was soon installed in a large, warm cage with her favourite toys and a caring nurse to look after her. Grateful for Sam's help, I went back home to shower and change my clothes before continuing my journey to the yard where the people were both understanding and accommodating. The horses were all worked up as the local hunt was in the area and their state of mind was similar to my own. Fortunately my usual calmness returned as soon as I started to work. I completely forgot my troubles; the horses settled down and the day went ahead as planned.

When I got home in the early evening, Dr Crowley returned my call and agreed with our plan to leave Rafiki in isolation for at least two days and bring her home when her faecal samples were clear. With any luck it could be as early as Saturday. That evening I donned a pair of rubber gloves and set about cleaning the floors, her bedding and all of the utility room and kitchen with an approved disinfectant to kill the bacteria. My friend Alison, a nurse, came to supper and we celebrated her promotion to Sister. The timing could not have been better as it was nice to relax and chat to someone who was a healthcare professional as well as a good friend.

The next morning I was up bright and early to give myself the first of the course of injections to stimulate my bone marrow. I was slightly apprehensive as I injected it under the skin of my abdomen but it was very straightforward and only momentarily uncomfortable. When the children left for school, I set off for the New Forest and enjoyed the drive in welcome sunshine. Donkeys and wild ponies grazed contentedly and I was lucky enough to see a stag standing stock still, silhouetted against the sun. I felt very positive as I knew Rafiki was in good hands and I was on my way to see a horse called Boss, who becomes grumpy when all is not well with his world. He is a small, handsome bay gelding who loves jumping and regularly comes home with a red rosette. From time to time, he strains a muscle or develops a sore back from his athletic endeavours and then he makes jolly sure we all know about it. Brushing him or changing his rugs becomes an exercise in avoiding the tossing head and gnashing teeth. His owners reach for the phone and summon me as part of their survival strategy.

What I particularly love about Boss is that although he swishes his tail and turns to bite as his rugs are removed, the minute I place my hands on him he quietens into a trance-like state. I gently feel his body with my fingers and although the individual muscles tense when I find the sore areas, Boss stays calm and lets me into his closely guarded space. As I insert the acupuncture needles, his head drops even lower and this deeply soporific state lasts for up to 30 minutes, giving me a chance to discuss his condition with the owners and catch up with their news as I only see them two or three times a year.

It was late morning by the time I finished treating Boss. As always it was a rewarding experience and I felt privileged to enjoy this mutually beneficial relationship with the feisty chap. However, throughout the morning I noticed that my tummy was exceptionally noisy and slightly unsettled. The weekend was coming up so perhaps I had better have a word with my GP in case I was brewing up for the same trouble as Rafiki. I missed catching Jane who had left the practice five minutes earlier but spoke to another nice lady doctor instead. She suggested I took a sample to the lab at the hospital and gave me some antibiotics in case I became unwell.

When I asked, 'How will I know if I have *Campylobacter?*' she replied, 'Explosive diarrhoea every hour, tummy ache, possibly vomiting and feeling poorly enough to go to bed.'

The next morning I had a phone call to say Rafiki was free of the infection and keen to come home. I, on the other hand, was not so good and this definitely looked like a case of shutting the stable door after the horse had bolted. Although I did not feel unwell, this was clearly no ordinary tummy upset. I managed to dash in and collect the puppy without mishap and she was overjoyed to be home. Shortly after that I was very touched when the kind doctor from the surgery telephoned to see how I was. She said she had been worrying about me and would not want to have a *Campylobacter* infection with a white cell count as low as mine. She recommended that I should start the antibiotics and contact the hospital if my symptoms became worse.

I suspect that vets can be annoying patients for doctors, as they do not always do as they are told. Certainly doctors can be frustrating clients for vets as they sometimes misdiagnose their pet's conditions and then treat them inappropriately. As I am allergic to penicillin and have a limited number of antibiotics available to me, I wanted to wait and see what happened next as I did not feel ill and we did not know for sure that I had

Campylobacter. The doctor warned me that as a vet I was likely to minimise the potential seriousness of my symptoms but reluctantly agreed that if that was the way I wanted to proceed then I must promise to take my pulse and temperature every hour and call her if I was worried.

My pulse at the time was 100 but I put that down to anxiety. I decided to read a book in the conservatory and promptly fell asleep. Two hours later I woke up feeling shivery and cold, despite wearing a warm coat under the duvet. My temperature was up so with gratitude I acknowledged that the doctor had been right all along. Thanks to her foresight in prescribing the antibiotics for me, I was able to start them straight away and by 11 p.m. my temperature had come back down to normal. Late that evening I went into Salisbury to collect Laura and her friend who had been to Truro for the day to represent Wilshire in the regional, cross-country running championships. This was undoubtedly one of those occasions when I should have stayed at home and asked friends to help as by now I felt pretty rough. It was nice, however, to greet the muddy, exhausted and happy girls as they had both qualified and would now represent the Southwest of England in the national finals. Their excitement was a real tonic.

The next morning was February 28th. I started the day outside in torrential rain, trying to unblock the outlet pipe to the natural pond in our front garden which was overflowing with rainwater from further up the village. The water was running across the driveway in sheets and flowing down the garden to collect in the dip outside the conservatory. It was now rising rapidly and within an inch of coming into the house. Thankfully I have a pump as this had happened once before so I could divert it out onto the road. Undoubtedly it was not wise to tackle this with a coat over my pyjamas when I was so unwell, but the task was urgent and at such an early hour on a

Sunday morning it seemed easier to get on with it, rather than trying to find someone else to help.

On that last day of February, I reached my lowest ebb. By the evening I felt overwhelmed with sadness as everyone seemed tired and tetchy and the boisterous puppy continually asked to play when I needed to rest. All I wanted at that moment was for someone to take over all my responsibilities and care for me.

HIGHS AND LOWS

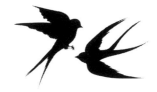

March 1ˢᵗ, the first day of spring! How quickly things can change. I woke up to brilliant sunshine and a hard, white frost which sparkled and glistened in the light. I was feeling much better and had injected myself and successfully flushed my line so that was a good start. The school bus did not turn up so our friend Stevie collected up the stranded children and drove them to Salisbury. It was his 50ᵗʰ birthday and he invited us to join him later for a party organised by his wife, Jacquie.

Later in the morning, the doctors confirmed that I had been infected with *Campylobacter*. To this day we do not know if Rafiki and I caught the disease from the many bird feeders in the garden as wild birds often excrete it, or whether she was a carrier anyway. From then on I fenced off the feeding stations so she could not hoover up any scattered seeds or bird droppings, and when refilling them each day I always wore rubber gloves and wellies that were subsequently dipped in disinfectant. I was reluctant to stop feeding the birds as they were a source of great pleasure and even now as I write, the blue tits and woodpeckers are enjoying the food just a few feet in front of me outside the window.

The day soon warmed up. All the wild crocuses opened in the small orchard under the ancient and wizened fruit trees at the side of our house. The carpet of snowdrops was still at its best and I spent a happy couple of hours capturing their beauty with my camera. The weather was so lovely that I stayed outside, raking up leaves and emptying the hanging baskets that were still in place from last summer. Rafiki played with the leaves and ran off with my gloves whenever I put them down.

In fact the whole week was unusually warm and sunny, a real joy for me as I had postponed working again until Friday. It gave me time to enjoy clearing the garden and catch up on outstanding jobs without feeling under pressure. There was time to remember my brother, Michael, who was born on March 3rd and sadly died unexpectedly aged just 40. It was also the day my dad died after a three-year struggle with leukaemia. He loved his garden and I often think of him when tending my own.

At 11 a.m. I put down my tools and walked down to the village hall for my first-ever visit to the Farley coffee morning, which takes place on the first Wednesday of every month. To my shame this is something I had never made time for when I was working full time and I discovered that for a pound, you are given a cup of tea or coffee, a choice of homemade cakes and a very warm welcome. It was an opportunity to catch up on the news and see some familiar faces as well as meet people who had recently moved into the village. When we arrived in Farley in 1987, we were made to feel welcome but it apparently caused quite a stir that outsiders had purchased the house. Nowadays the situation is completely different, with properties changing hands more frequently. Two ladies who did not know I was wearing a wig commented favourably on my new haircut which made me smile. Most people were aware of my situation as I found it easier that way and never made it a secret. There was another lady present who been through it all herself a couple of years earlier and she was particularly kind.

By Friday I was recovered enough to go back to work and enjoyed another day in the New Forest. I called in to have lunch and a chat with my friend Tim, a dairy farmer, and was sorry not to be able to introduce Rafiki, who was still in quarantine, to his yellow Labrador, Boris. I also enjoyed a visit to the nearby farm shop and bought some primroses to plant in the garden at the weekend.

The following day I had an upsetting and unfortunate experience. A friend had arrived with his chainsaw to cut up a fallen tree and we had a blazing bonfire to burn all the twigs. I was enjoying myself immensely until I realised I had melted my precious wig. I had been warned not to expose it to the blast of heat when opening the door of a hot oven, but I thought I had kept a sufficient distance from the flames. At that moment I understood how important it had become to me and felt its loss acutely. In the afternoon I spent hours painstakingly trimming the singed ends off thousands of individual hairs, which improved it a little but not enough. I knew it was one of the Raquel Welch 'Signature Collection' so I searched on the Internet and was lucky enough to find a possible supplier. On Monday morning after an agonizing wait, I received a phone call confirming that it was in stock. The replacement arrived three days later, slightly blonder than the original, but nevertheless very welcome.

* * *

The following week was one of ups and downs. Kitkat, our black and white cat, now developed a high temperature and acute diarrhoea. As I took him into the vet's to be kept in isolation and prevent him contaminating the house further, I wondered when this was all going to end.

Later that day the Godolphin School Under 15 lacrosse team won the National Schools Championships, to add to the gold medal won by their senior team. This was the first time any school had achieved double success and we were very proud to see both teams on the regional section of the 6 o'clock news. Laura played for the Under 15s, so it was wonderful to have something so exciting to celebrate.

By then I had been sufficiently subdued by recent events to listen to my body and respond accordingly. I spaced my work out and did a little less. It had become a necessity to take great care to avoid any further infections and there were days when I just stayed at home and rested as I acknowledged how tired I was.

I cannot remember which nurse gave me my fourth round of chemotherapy as I have nothing written in my diary for that or the next couple of days. I think this reflected my energy levels despite having an encouragingly improved white cell count. I know I moaned to the children that they were lazy and inconsiderate; they in turn remember me being tetchy and intolerant so the truth was probably somewhere in between. Some of my diary entries just say 'Tired, tired, tired'.

I was able to take on selected new clients and treating their horses together with my regular patients gave me the energy boost I needed. I forgot my troubles and enjoyed helping to resolve theirs. My friends continued to look after me. Rosie, a complementary therapist, treated my weary body to hot stone massages and sent me a text every day. Wendy, my fellow veterinary acupuncturist friend, drove up from Devon to keep me company at Somerley horse trials where we enjoyed watching our patients perform, despite bitterly cold and wet weather. Alex and Laura were marvellous with the way they coped. They hugged me every day, told me I looked nice when I made the effort to dress up and outwardly carried on as normal —a remarkable feat with Laura at a relatively new school and Alex doing his A levels. How lucky I was!

49

APRIL AT LAST

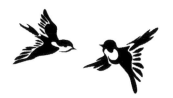

I have always loved April. I associate it with spring, my favourite colour yellow and my birthday. And by the end of the month the treatment would be over (or so I thought). At last!

On April 1st I reported to the Pembroke Suite for my blood test (which was fine) and then bothered Dr Crowley with several questions. It always amazed me that she could read my list upside down from the other side of the room and keep one step ahead of me. This time I queried her decision not to give me radiotherapy after all and she confirmed that there was a sufficient margin of normal tissue around my tumour for her to consider that radiotherapy was not necessary. That was a very welcome reprieve.

Easter weekend was most enjoyable and Anne arrived on Monday evening to accompany me to my fifth chemotherapy. I was pleased to have her there because I woke up on Tuesday morning feeling sick. I had now developed anticipatory nausea and the thought of the Pembroke Suite and its characteristic smell turned my stomach. The image of the red epirubicin being injected into the drip tube was the worst trigger but once I got there, I was fine. This time Sally, who normally worked in the next-door Pembroke Ward where the cancer inpatients are cared for, looked after me. During the treatment Anne and I chatted to a friendly lady in the next bed who told us about the ghastly side-effects she had experienced after each treatment. Once again I appreciated how lucky I had been.

The next day it was back to the vet with Rafiki who was diagnosed with yet another chronic problem. Poor little thing. I could have done without the expense and the worry but it certainly stopped me brooding about myself. I had to smile when the children said that next time I picked a puppy out of a litter they would make sure we came away with a different one.

Then it was back to work and delightful for me as the owners of the lovely horse I went to see next were not only nice but had eight golden retrievers. A Spanish vet joined me who had the same acupuncture qualifications as me but wanted to improve her English and practical equine skills. She was very knowledgeable and good at examining the horses, so I enjoyed her company and challenging questions. We were pleased because after his first acupuncture treatment seven days earlier, the persistent diarrhoea that the horse had experienced for the previous six months had instantly stopped. His tail and hind limbs that had been dirty and soaking wet were now completely dry and he was reported to be more comfortable and happier in himself.

April was an interesting mix of good days and very tired days, but the approach of my final treatment mentally spurred me on. Throughout the whole cancer experience, I felt the need particularly to enjoy any special occasions and that included my birthday. On April 15th I woke up with Laura snuggled up beside me and bright sunshine outside. Over breakfast I opened my presents which included a book from Alex and a pretty Indian top from Laura. On the kitchen table was a coffee cake covered with sugar-coated, speckled chocolate eggs which Laura had made after I went to bed the previous evening. A lovely start to the day and in the evening we went to my favourite Indian restaurant with Izzy, Katie and Meg.

I completed and enjoyed another week at work and generally celebrated that I had experienced so few of the many possible side-effects. Then on the 21st April, just four days before the sixth and final chemotherapy, I woke up and realised that my chest felt sore. As I undid my pyjama top, I found a grape-sized swelling around the exit site of my Groshong line. Was this harmless oedema or cellulitis caused by infection? I was due to travel quite a distance to see a horse in Reigate that day and was reluctant to change my plans. After a few minutes of gentle massage and moving my arm around to get the circulation going, I reluctantly decided to start the day with an unscheduled trip to the Pembroke Suite. I hoped that if I turned up first thing, someone would glance at the swelling, give me antibiotics and allow me to escape.

The reality of course was somewhat different. The wonderful staff of the Pembroke Suite swung into action and took it all far more seriously than I did. I was shown into a side room where a nurse took my temperature and pulse then asked me what had happened to cause my rather low blood pressure. She took a blood sample and sent it to the lab for culture as well as the usual tests for red and white cell counts and liver and kidney function. After a short wait, I met Phillipa, a young doctor, for the first time. She was kind and gentle in her examination and prescribed some antibiotics for me. Then I was monitored for another couple of hours before being allowed to leave.

As I felt fine in myself, I just switched my work around and went to treat a local horse instead. That was a most enjoyable experience as it gave me a chance to catch up with Kirsty, the policewoman owner of a lovely fifteen-year-old mare called Millie. I noticed, though, that as I stretched my right arm, my chest became increasingly tender. By the time I got home, the infection had tracked along the tube under my skin and the swelling was now the shape and size of a small pear. Oops. In retrospect perhaps I should have stayed at home and I now felt anxious and fragile. The antibiotics needed a chance to work. When I phoned the hospital, the nurse advised me to monitor my temperature during the evening and go in for intravenous antibiotics if it started to rise.

By 9:30 a.m. the next day, I was back in the Pembroke Suite. My temperature was fine and I felt back to normal. If anything, the infection was slightly less hot and painful, but it had spread across the entire right side of my chest wall and there was a discharge leaking around the line. The nurses and doctors were sympathetic and we discussed whether to remove the line now or try and leave it in for the last treatment. I was keen to get rid of it but they decided to start intravenous antibiotics and review the situation the following day.

It was later that afternoon that I made a silly mistake. I sat out in the late afternoon sun and soaked up its warm rays for a most enjoyable half hour. There was a cool breeze so I wore a coat as I faced the setting sun. All chemotherapy patients are advised not to sunbathe as the skin is more likely to burn and I did not realise how sensitive my normally sun-tolerant skin was. I was wearing a V-necked sweatshirt and the exposed areas of my face and chest became decidedly pink. I was so cross with myself for not thinking and taking more care.

By the following morning, the infected area had definitely improved and was better still by the afternoon. The nurses gave me more intravenous antibiotics at the hospital and took blood to check that I was fit for Monday's chemotherapy. Over the weekend I continued with intravenous and oral antibiotics. The infection subsided and although I did not feel unwell, my energy levels sank. I just about made it into Salisbury for my Saturday coffee with Izzy, which cheered me up as the children were away for the weekend.

On Sunday a friend came and mowed the lawn for me. The garden looked very pretty with spring flowers and I sat outside, huddled up in a coat hoping for some sun and some energy but neither came. In the evening, however, cousin Anne arrived and brightened up the day. She brought champagne and yellow roses —my favourite treats.

Since I did not drink alcohol during the week of my treatment and she could only stay a couple of days, we opened the bottle and made our usual toast to health and happiness.

On Monday the 26th April, my last chemotherapy went ahead and then the line came out—what a relief! In a couple of days, I would at last be able to submerge myself in a lovely warm, deep bath. A bacterium called *Moraxella catarrhalis* had been grown from swabs taken the previous week and the line was later confirmed as the source of the infection. That meant I had to continue daily visits to the hospital for treatment and I also had an ECG and echocardiogram. I had noticed that my legs had some fluid retention and I felt bloated—more than the seven pounds of weight gain. I think my poor heart and body were struggling to cope with all the medication.

I am sure there are sound medical reasons for limiting the chemotherapy to six treatments but mentally and physically I had had enough. For the first time, I stayed quietly resting at home all week to be fit enough for a trip to Badminton Horse Trials on Friday.

50

THE END OF TREATMENT

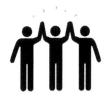

After the week of attending the hospital for antibiotics and check-ups, I was given the OK to go to Badminton. This is one of the highlights of my year and one I traditionally attend with my friend Rosie. I have been fortunate enough to be involved in the preparation of a number of horses for this test of athleticism, ability and stamina that takes place over three days and that year was no exception. I was obviously not up to walking the four-mile cross-country course on the Saturday along with the other 220,000 spectators, so we went on Friday to watch some dressage and go shopping. The hundreds of trade stands are an important feature of Badminton where you can buy everything a horse and rider could possibly need along with a wide range of other goods from dog accessories to designer clothing and jewellery.

We left at 6:30 a.m. and arrived a couple of hours later to find patchy sunshine and a chilly breeze. A brisk walk around part of the cross-country course and a hot drink warmed us up before some serious spending with the credit card. My favourite but most self-indulgent purchase was some dangly earrings with pink and green semi-precious stones that were very pretty.

Having a friend to encourage the purchase and say you deserve it always helps to ease the conscience! The next success was a cheap but stylish waterproof hat from the menswear stall to protect my wig from the intermittent rain. We met up with friends to share our picnics and watch the dressage. All in all a most enjoyable time, made more exciting by one of my clients ending the day in a very satisfactory position on the scoreboard.

When I got home and sat down, I noticed that despite the exercise, the elastic of my socks had made deep indentations in my heavy-feeling legs. I finished the last of my routine, post-chemo medication and the antibiotics that night and heaved a sigh of relief. The following evening, I had eaten supper and was watching TV when my tummy seemed to expand in front of my eyes. I was resigned to the weight gain, but this was something else. When I got undressed, I was horrified to find accumulations of subcutaneous fluid hanging down from my abdomen and the tops of my thighs like wobbly jellies. Unfortunately it was now past 11 p.m. and too late to feel comfortable about disturbing any of my doctor friends. Feeling more than a little scared, I went to bed and just as I was dropping off to sleep became alarmed by strange noises, only to realise it was me snoring. It seemed that even my nasal passages and soft palate were becoming congested. I wondered if my low blood pressure was contributing to these unexpected symptoms.

The next morning the swelling was no worse but I felt a bit odd so Rosie came over with Alice her Labrador to keep me company and watch the cross-country phase of Badminton Horse Trials on TV. It was a chilly day so after letting the dogs play in the field, I lit a log fire in the lounge and we settled down to watch the action. Rosie was marvellous—she brought the lunch with her and refused to let me do anything. By early afternoon though I was clearly not well. Waves of blackness washed over me and I came close to passing out. Five minutes after each episode, I was back to normal and still able to enjoy the day.

I did not phone the Pembroke Ward as I was concerned they would ask me to come in and I did not want to put other poorly cancer patients at risk of catching anything from me. It was also the weekend and as I was not an emergency, I would probably have to wait some time to see a doctor. Rosie offered to stay the night but Alex and Laura came home from their dad's house to be with me, which was very comforting.

By the next day, I was more or less back to normal. Goodness knows what it was all about but the swelling had gone and I was much better. It felt as though my body had begun to rid itself of the toxic medication once and for all. A day or two afterwards, I developed a ghastly thrush infection in my mouth and throat and as soon as that had cleared up, I woke up with conjunctivitis. Whatever next? Some of my fellow patients experienced nasty infections after every treatment so once again I realised how lucky I had been. Thank goodness it was all over.

51

LIGHT ON THE HORIZON

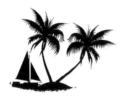

Mᴀy was a month of new beginnings and gentle recovery. I had to pace myself and work three days a week, feeling full of energy on the days I treated horses and quietly tired on the other days. To all of my lovely clients—you know who you are—I thank you for taking care of me and having faith in my ability to continue treating your special and precious horses. Carrying on with work gave me the confidence and strength to overcome little health hiccups along the way and made me feel valued.

I had a new challenge too. With Alex and Laura, I registered to take part in the Walk for Wards, which is one of the Stars Appeal charity events to raise money for Salisbury District Hospital. I wanted to give something back towards the cost of the excellent care I had received and to say thank you to the doctors and nurses of the Breast Care Department and the Pembroke Suite. With the support of Dave in the Stars Appeal office, I set up a Just Giving online fundraising page and armed with their posters and collection boxes, I made a giant notice board and placed it prominently in my driveway. The donations came in steadily and I updated the total on the board each week. The generosity of my friends, family and the people of Farley was heart-warming. There was a choice of three-kilometre and ten-kilometre walks and I elected to enjoy every step of the shorter route, rather than risk overdoing it.

Although the treatment was over, seeing yourself in the mirror is a permanent reminder of the cancer. You want to celebrate and be normal but have to be patient. My hair began to reappear before the last chemotherapy as a dark shadow with frosty white tips—in other words completely grey. That was another blow to my confidence, albeit a temporary one as it soon reverted to mostly brown. Although I loved my wig and was grateful for it, there were days when I felt like childishly screaming, 'But I don't want to wear a wig,' when someone gave me a compliment. I will not forget the response of a dear friend who had not seen me for a while. 'Gosh, you do look tired,' she said as I got out of the car to treat her horse. Then, 'No you don't; you just look older,' which was absolutely true.

At the beginning of May, I planted a wildflower garden with seed I had purchased the previous year. Rafiki eventually had to be shut indoors as she kept attacking the gardening fork. She was particularly fond of fighting with garden tools, brooms and for some reason the pole that held up the washing line. Once the pole had succumbed and was on the floor, she pulled on the sheets and duvet covers with such force that the branch of the tree that the line was attached to came down as well. All part of the fun in a Labrador puppy's day. Her behaviour at home may not have been helpful but at work she was still a very good pup and sat quietly on her mat, enjoying the days out.

Yet again my friends were an important feature in this period of recovery. My friend Rod, who lives in Malaysia and is Alex's godfather, came to stay for a couple of days. I have known Rod since university days and his easy company was relaxing and restorative for all of us. Then I met my friend Sara at the O2 for a much-looked-forward-to Westlife concert. I was expecting us to have a coffee and sandwich first but just as my train pulled into Waterloo station I received a text inviting me for a drink in an Argentinean restaurant before the performance.

I had never taken much notice of the numerous places to eat at the O2 but found myself in a very elegant setting where everything was black, white and silver, including the smartly attired waiters and waitresses. In the subdued light, I could see Sara waving from a circular, sunken area of the bar, sipping champagne and nibbling smoky bacon-flavoured popcorn. What a welcome! She was on sparkling form and after we moved upstairs and selected from a choice of steaks that were brought to our table for viewing, she told me that this amazing meal was her treat to celebrate the end of my treatment. The whole experience is now a treasured memory that I shall never forget.

My favourite music could always be relied upon to lift my mood and I confess to being a fan of boy bands including Boyzone, Cold Play, Westlife and Take That, together with opera-style singers such as Russell Watson and Katherine Jenkins. I was lucky enough to enjoy several live concerts and as they were always booked well in advance, reaching them represented another step forward in either my treatment or recovery.

In the middle of May, I had a scare because my sternum and ribs close to the surgical site became very painful. Perhaps understandably I was afraid that the cancer had returned and was grateful to Dr Crowley for her reassurance and for arranging an ultrasound scan that put my mind at rest. At this time, however, my body often hurt. Gardening and planting out the bedding meant that the pots and tubs provided a riot of colour but came at a cost as I sometimes overdid things and strained my weakened muscles. Thank heavens for Jenny, my chiropractor friend, who came to my rescue and patched me up time after time. Towards the end of May, I realised that if I wanted to continue working, I needed to rest all weekend as I was very, very tired.

52

SUMMER ARRIVES

I find it fascinating that my memory can be so selective. If you asked me how the summer was, I would reply that it was wonderful, remembering only the good bits, of which there were many. Looking back through my diaries though, there were also times when I felt frustrated and grumpy because I was simply too tired to get on top of the jobs that needed doing. Recovery was a slow process and on occasions I felt the effort of getting well, looking after a family and running my own business to be an almost overwhelming responsibility. Sometimes I felt anxious and did not know why but thanks to my natural resilience and the continuing help from my friends, family and Sarah in the Psychology department, I came through those difficult times.

One of the highlights was the sponsored Walk for Wards. In the preceding weeks, the *Salisbury Journal* ran several features on the participants with their individual stories. I was happy to be included but when someone from Wiltshire Radio telephoned to ask if I would do an interview, my shyness got the better of me and I said I needed to think about it. As the day went on, I decided this was a good time to get over it and to promote the worthwhile event. I met a kindly presenter from Wilshire Radio at a café in Wilton and did two separate interviews, one of which was used in a later feature.

The 20th June was bright and sunny, the perfect weather for a walk. Alex, Laura and I dressed in our Stars Appeal T-shirts and sat down to breakfast with the radio on. I was kept in suspense as the presenter did an amazing job of building up my story.

'She found a lump and knew it was cancer,' he said then followed up with, 'Coming up is an inspirational story of a Wiltshire woman. Sue Devereux will be with us later.'

I was on the edge of my seat, wondering what Sue Devereux would sound like and was going to say. I need not have worried as the interview had been edited well and paid tribute to the hospital where I had received so much good care.

The walk took place in the grounds of Wilton House, a venue that features in many of my happy memories. When the previous Lord Pembroke was alive, I took care of the veterinary needs of the horses and ponies on the estate. It was a good place to work and when the children's adventure playground opened, we were amongst the first to support it with an annual membership. There were picnics and ice creams by the river and the pleasure of enjoying the beautiful house and gardens. We regularly attended the July concerts and fireworks that made for magical evenings with our friends.

The atmosphere was an upbeat and happy one and before the start, we made signs to wear on our backs, stating which ward we were supporting. Then the crowds lined up in front of the house, ready for the off. There were babies in buggies, young children and adults representing the whole spectrum from the young to the elderly. Reading the labels on people's backs was often touching. For part of the walk I removed my wig and enjoyed the feeling of cool air on my head as we passed through parts of the estate I had not visited before. We were given a big cheer and a medal as we crossed the finish line and had our photo taken which later appeared in *Salisbury Life* magazine. Then there was lunch and free ice cream and a chance to chat with the other participants. Alex and Laura were good company and entered the spirit of the day; between us we raised £1,500.

* * *

In July my work with the event horses continued and then owners asked me to examine some of the top dressage horses. When my work took me further afield, I made the appointments for a Friday when it was the children's weekend with their father. That way I was under no pressure to get home and often combined the trip with an evening and overnight stop with a friend in the area. So it was that Liz and I spent a delightful evening reminiscing in her garden with a bar-b-q and bottle of wine as the sun went down.

With some reservations I allowed Laura to camp with her friends at the Larmer Tree Festival under Alex's supervision. This is a local event with a magical mix of entertainment for all ages including music, comedy, theatre and art, along with delicious and unusual food. As she was just fifteen years old, I was worried about letting her attend, but it was a great success and I discovered a safe and happy atmosphere when I joined them one evening. I purchased some colourful bandanas to wear with or instead of my wig and enjoyed the music despite the rain.

Towards the end of July, we shared a family day out in London. We wanted to see Russ Abbot playing Fagin in the musical *Oliver*, as he is the brother of our friend Don and we had met him on several occasions. With the family railcard, we bought train tickets to London and went for lunch in Covent Garden. I will not forget my mistake of agreeing to walk up the stairs from the Underground instead of waiting for the lift. The 193 steps seemed never-ending, and I was breathless and speechless by the time I reached the top. Minutes earlier on the Tube, I had been very touched when a lady caught my eye and asked if I would like her seat. It was the first day I had left my wig at home and was declaring to myself and the world that I was back to normal. Her kindness and the steps showed me that I was kidding myself and the fine covering of downy hair on my head was a definite giveaway.

* * *

The goal that kept me going was the thought of our holiday in Turkey with Izzy, Katie and Meg. When the time finally arrived, we flew from Bournemouth Airport to Dalyan and I felt a wave of relaxation as the warm air surrounded us as the top of the aircraft steps. By 4 p.m. we were sitting by the pool enjoying the late afternoon sun at the Hotel Yunus. It was 28°C with a light breeze, and crickets singing in the background. With the gentle chug of motor cruisers passing by on the river and happy sounds of children playing and people talking, I lay back on the sunbed and soaked up the warmth.

The days began with a swim in the warm pool before a delicious breakfast of fresh bread, fruit and cheeses eaten on a wooden veranda that extended over the river in the shade of fig trees and clumps of bamboo. Little birds hovered to collect any crumbs and terrapins gathered hopefully with open mouths in the water below. Most days we sat and read books in the gardens or by the pool with occasional sightseeing or early morning trips to see kingfishers and turtles. The colourful Saturday markets were always fun with the vendors assuring us they were 'very good fakes'. In the evenings we walked the kilometre into the town and enjoyed some memorable and happy family meals. Sometimes we ate by the harbour and sometimes we spent the evening in the market square near the mosque or along the main shopping street.

Wherever we went the Turkish people were always friendly and hospitable.

I believe that my recovery really began in Turkey. After months of not being able to get to sleep, I found myself drifting off in the morning, the afternoon and again at night. It was a lovely feeling and by the time we came home in mid-August, I felt mentally and physically refreshed. There was more good news when Alex learnt he had achieved the A-level grades required for a place at Cardiff, his first choice of university.

At the end of the month, I flew to Denmark for the International Veterinary Acupuncture Society Annual Congress with my friend Wendy. Vets from all over the world who practise acupuncture meet up to share their ideas and experience. Friendships are made and there is a wide variety of lectures and practical classes to choose from. We looked forward to listening to our colleague Thomas who somehow makes complex neurophysiology into a fascinating story—we were not disappointed—and to Kerry, a very experienced equine vet, acupuncturist and chiropractor from South Carolina.

I first heard Kerry lecture when I began studying acupuncture in 1999. The course was intense and I struggled to grasp some of the concepts of Traditional Chinese Medicine at that stage. Then Kerry started to speak with such insight and wisdom about examining and treating horses that I was completely spellbound as pearls of wisdom flowed from the mouth of this tall and gentle man. In Denmark he demonstrated some simple chiropractic techniques and achieved excellent results on an initially fractious mare that quickly relaxed in his hands. As soon as we were back home, I tried them on several event horses that were bound for Burghley and Blenheim Horse Trials and was delighted to find they worked for me too. I have always thought that if attending a conference changes just one aspect of my work for the better, then it was worthwhile. It is with thanks to Kerry that I was sufficiently inspired to register for the International Academy of Veterinary Chiropractic course, starting in March 2011.

So the future looked bright, interesting and positive. I can look back on that year and see that at times I made some unwise decisions and probably pushed myself too hard. All very well in hindsight but as a chemotherapy patient you do whatever you have to to get through it, a day at a time. I preferred not to think about the cancer which was probably why I hated seeing myself in the mirror. Now I happily ruffle the new mop of brown curls that have taken the place of my wig.

And the experience was not all bad either. I feel a stronger person having let go of some of the thought patterns that previously constrained me. I know what really matters and who my friends are. I no longer strive for impossible goals and have learnt to appreciate the present rather than always planning the future.

53

MOVING ON

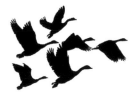

The summer drew to its end and I had a great deal to be thankful for. There had been a deluge of rain over the last few days but the sun finally came out on this particular morning. Water was dripping from the trees that were beginning to lose their brown and yellow leaves, and the air was humid and warm.

The previous night I slept well with a wide-open window, listening to the rain and feeling the gentle breeze. With a gloomy weather forecast for the next week, I walked Rafiki around the village. It felt good to be part of a caring community and we stopped for a chat with a number of different people. How I love the warmth of late summer with hints of autumn all round. I walked slowly, willing summer to last a little longer.

We passed through green fields with young beef cattle on the horizon. The hedgerows were laden with ripe blackberries and small white butterflies danced above the long grass. I felt quite tired but inspired to keep walking by the boundless energy of my young Labrador. She is so full of joy and fun.

As I climbed over the rickety gate and back onto the road, I came to our beautiful church and decided to call in to sit and think. The sound of organ music escaped through the open doorway so not wanting to disturb whoever was playing, I walked around the church into the graveyard behind with my thoughts. I passed through a gap in the tumbledown wall under the shade of yew and horse chestnut trees and entered a small, sunny, enclosed area. As I read the names on the gravestones, I remembered those who were no longer with us, many of whom were my friends. Had I really lived in Farley for 23 years?

I sat on a wooden bench in the warm sun and soaked up the familiar sights and sounds. In front of me a large and elegant copper beech tree with low-spreading branches blocked most of my view of the church. An apple tree on my left was laden with fruit which was dropping onto the ground below. To my right a tall hedge separated the engraved stones that were surrounded by wild flowers from the farmland beyond.

When I closed my eyes, I could hear birdsong and the sound of happy children playing. It was warm and I felt content. The puppy sat quietly at my feet. Like the seasons, nothing in life is constant or to be taken for granted. I have always said that I want my final resting place to be there; it was so peaceful and surrounded by beauty that remains unspoilt with the passage of time.

But my time had not yet come. I still had plenty to do and planned to make a full recovery. Before the gathering storm clouds hid the sunlight, I stroked my young dog and we walked out of the churchyard to meet the future. My future. With many more stories to tell.

MESSAGE FROM THE AUTHOR

I sincerely thank you for reading my story. If you enjoyed it, I would be grateful if you could leave a review on Amazon. More information about the Salisbury District Hospital Stars Appeal Charity can be found on www.starsappeal.org

For those of you who enjoy reading memoirs I recommend you look at the Facebook group We Love Memoirs, www.facebook.com/groups/welovememoirs

ABOUT THE AUTHOR

Sue Devereux qualified as a vet at Bristol University in 1983 and started her veterinary career in a mixed practice in Wimborne, Dorset, where she treated a wide variety of animals, embracing the challenges with enthusiasm. Subsequently she went on to establish her own practice, treating horses and ponies with acupuncture and chiropractic when they did not respond to conventional treatment.

Sue has two grown-up children and enjoys riding and competing her horse in local show jumping competitions. In 2009 Sue was diagnosed with breast cancer and underwent surgery and chemotherapy, with a further episode in 2017.

Now fully recovered, Sue continues to work as a vet and enjoys writing and spending time with her friends and family. She lives in the village of Farley with her two horses, a yellow Labrador, a golden retriever and two tabby cats.

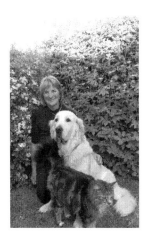

ACKNOWLEDGEMENTS

I would like to thank Jacky Donovan and Victoria Twead at Ant Press for guiding me through the publishing process and bringing the book to life. Thanks must also go to Maggie Raynor and Judy Linard for designing the cover. Finally I would like to thank all of my friends, family, clients and patients who are included in the book, together with those who encouraged me to tell my story.

Printed in Great Britain
by Amazon